Pregnancy Yog.

with Laurence Turner

Pregnancy Yoga
with Laurence Turner

Disclaimer

Not all pregnancy Yoga exercises are suitable for everyone and this or any exercise programme may result in injury. Consult with your doctor before you exercise.

To reduce the risk of injury it is important not to force or strain yourself during exercise. If you feel pain, stop and seek medical attention if necessary.

Pregnant women should not perform abdominal twists, bends or tightening exercises. Those with special health considerations should consult their medical practitioner before performing any exercise.

The creators, producers, performers of Yogamoo cannot guarantee this product is suitable and safe for every individual.

Any liability, loss or damage in connection with the use of Yogamoo information or Pregnancy-yoga.net and its Yoga instruction, including but not limited to any liability, loss or damage arising from the performance of the exercises demonstrated here, or any advice or information provided by Laurence Turner, practice in the videos, or on the website, is expressly disclaimed.

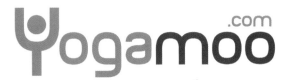

First Published in Great Britain in 2010 by Yogamoo

Copyright – Yogamoo

ISBN-13:978-1453709382
ISBN-10:145370938X

Contents

Foreword

I hope this book will inspire you to practice whether attending classes or practicing from home using specialist material.

Enjoy this special time.

Here is a basic synopsis of what Yoga can do for you in pregnancy. Students commonly think of Yoga in terms of fitness and relaxation; it is but also much more. During pregnancy senses are heightened mostly because of the enormous amount of blood that circulates in your veins, subtly affecting your own internal rhythm or body clock and in turn your notion of time.

Because of this you are more susceptible to experience the real benefits of Yoga, being able to experience the unity of mind, body and soul through the breath and the sense of relaxation and detachment that comes with it.

Of course, Yoga does aim to make you birth fit. A lot of the postures are designed to build strength and stamina ahead of labour as well as alleviate pregnancy ailments.

Pregnancy Yoga will also help with mental and emotional preparation for the birth and for having your baby. These aspects are usually not dealt with by physical disciplines. Yoga will provide instant access to Relaxation through your practice of Breathing techniques; this will be of paramount important on the day of the birth.

The Meditation aspect of Yoga will help to quieten the mind and help you dissociate from overwhelming sensations in labour.

With practice, you will build the confidence that your body knows how to deliver your baby in the same manner that it knew how to conceive and knows how to be pregnant.

This confidence and access to deep Relaxation will help you be more in control of your birth while you surrender to the power of nature. The physical discomforts will be lessened.

As for the emotional bond, Yoga offers you to share this quiet time for yourself with your unborn child and perhaps already get to know each other through the exchange of positive and joyful thoughts, sounds and love.

About Laurence

Yogamoo and Pregnancy Yoga are owned and run by Laurence Turner. Yogamoo teaches Pregnancy Yoga classes in Redhill and Reigate in Surrey near London in the United Kingdom.

Laurence Turner is a French National. She lived in France until she graduated from Lille Business School. Laurence moved over to the UK and lived in South London while taking a Master Degree in Foreign Affairs at the University of Westminster in Regent Street.

Laurence likes eating great food in nice restaurants and relaxing in the garden. She loves skiing and swimming and meeting friends.

Her ambition was to work for the United Nations however she took her first job with a global leader in electronic components trading and spent 2 years at their Headquarters in Montreal. Laurence transferred to the London branch and pursued a career in the electronics and IT industry in sales, product marketing and supply chain positions.

She has been interested in health and sports since her late teens when she started swimming on a weekly basis. She subsequently used the local gyms, started jogging and joined the local Tae Kwan Do club. She continued Tae Kwan Do while living in Montreal and studied T'ai Chi there during 2 years with Master Sergio Arione.

Back in England, she was looking to resume a martial art class however did not seem to find the right school. She went travelling around the world in 2001 when she met Phillip her husband-to-be in Australia. However she didn't encounter Yoga until her return to England in 2002 at the Wandsworth Virgin gym.

There she had found what she had been looking for and enrolled herself with various teachers and classes several times a week. She attended courses, retreats and several Yoga and Meditation workshops in South London, some of which were based at the Putney Sivananda Centre and at that time became aware of their Teachers Training Programme.

She married Phillip in the South of France and they moved to Reigate, Surrey where Laurence's office was based. Laurence continued to study and practice Yoga with Instructor Brenda Brown attaining a Yoga Alliance recognised Diploma. A little while after the birth of their daughter Luz, Laurence decided to qualify to teach Pregnancy Yoga and Children Yoga.

Laurence's passion for helping people and her calm nature through empathy allows her to fulfil her lifelong dream to enable individuals to succeed and progress in both mind and body.

Introduction

This manual aims to provide you with the necessary knowledge to help you put together routines that you can practice at home. In Chapter I you will learn the benefits associated with the group of postures that are helpful in Pregnancy Yoga. In Chapter II a number of sequences from each group have been designed for you to build a varied and suitable home practice. All you need is to set aside 20-60 minutes once or several times a week and a small space for a Yoga mat. The sequence builder on page 48 makes it so easy to use.

In addition, the benefits of Pregnancy Yoga are not restricted to physical fitness and stamina. There are mental and emotional benefits also that will help prepare you for labour and for welcoming your baby. In Chapter I you will learn how Breathing and Relaxation techniques can focus your mind and relax your body, both critical tools for labour and for daily life after the birth. In Chapter III a series of guided Relaxation practices has been included along with Relaxation postures for you to practice.

In your first trimester, it is generally recommended to slow down your practice as your body is going through tremendous changes. It is a good time to focus on your Breathing, Relaxation and Meditation practice with few physical postures, preferably from the Warming or Calming routines on page 48. In your second and third trimesters, once your hormones have stabilized, your pregnancy is well established and your energy levels increase, you can start a more physical practice including sequences from the Energising or Complete routines on page 48. Be sure to listen to your body and take plenty of rest as needed.

As you become familiar with the postures, the Breathing and the Relaxation practices of Yoga they will prepare you effectively for labour. The skills you learn now will also be helpful in postnatal and in everyday life in the future. I wish you all the very best in your practice.

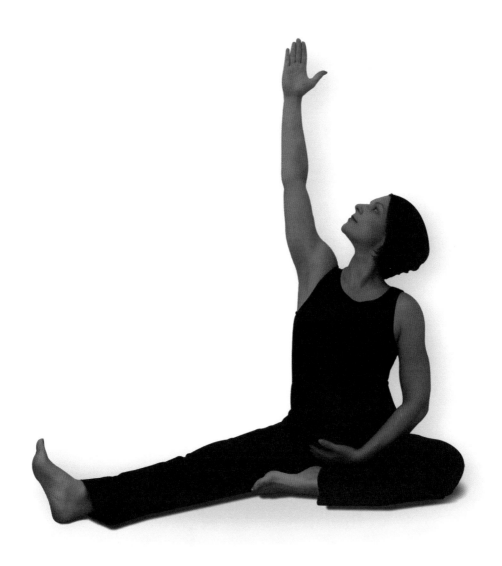

Chapter I
Why Yoga in Pregnancy

Yoga for Pregnancy: Physical Benefits and Practice

There are many ways to practice Yoga. I always encourage my students to tune in to how they feel at the time they have set for practice, with the intention of giving their body what it needs at that time. You may practice any sequences of any group of postures as long as you take a few minutes to prepare and finish.

If you have time for a complete practice then I would encourage you to start with a Breathing Exercise, then Seated postures and All Fours postures, followed by Standing postures, Final Floor postures and Relaxation. Practiced in that order, the sequences will gently bring your body up from seated position to standing and progressively warming all the muscles and joints in the body.

As a rule, a practice bringing heat in the body is always followed by a cooling down sequence which will help slow you down gently, stretch the muscles and prepare you for the final Relaxation. A Yoga practice starts with a Breathing Exercise which helps calm and centre yourself and finishes with a Relaxation period, often lying down propped up or on your left-side to allow yourself and your body to rest and recuperate fully.

Should you only want to practice Relaxation today, this is absolutely fine. Start with whatever sequence you intuitively feel like practicing at that moment in time. This is an ideal way to build your personal practice.

In the following section you will learn the benefits of each group of postures to guide you in your practice.

What Postures to Practice

Seated Postures

These postures can be practiced all the way through your pregnancy. If you are suffering from pelvic pain and in particular Symphysis Pubis Dysfunction or SPD keep your knees in front of your hips at all times and avoid taking the knees out wide.

Seated postures are a great way to start your practice with a few minutes in a simple cross-legged position when you can practice some Meditative Breathing and follow with some arm movements to loosen up the shoulders and gently warm up.

Arm Stretches and Simple Open Twists will provide a wonderful warm up for the spine. As you stretch up you will offer more space for your abdominal organs which may relieve heart burn, a common ailment in pregnancy.

As you stretch up through the arms and open up underneath the armpits, this stimulates the lymphatic system around the axillary lymph nodes, a very beneficial practice ahead of breast-feeding and for general breast tissue health.

Leg position can be changed from cross-legged to Butterfly Pose with the soles of the feet together to practice opening the hips, a gentle way to keep the pelvis mobile and flexible ahead of labour.

As you extend one leg out into a One Leg Forward Bend position you will stretch the back of the legs, hamstrings and calves. This will help if you suffer from leg cramps at night.

All Fours Postures

These postures can be practiced all the way through your pregnancy even when suffering from the SPD front pelvic pain, in which case keep both knees or feet on the floor.

Postures on All Fours are an essential part of a Yoga practice. There are countless variations that help stretch and move the spine, strengthen the arms, wrists and shoulders, an essential foundation for other Yoga poses.

In pregnancy these postures are also used in preparation for labour and to provide more space for your baby especially if you have been sitting at a desk all day or sitting in a car. The posture with the help of gravity encourages your abdominal organs to regain their place and offers more space for your baby to turn to its optimum foetal position.

Simple Cat Stretches and their variations will help keep the spine mobile and healthy. As you round the spine in an arch keep moving with the flow of the breath for an energising and meditative practice.

You can also move forwards and backwards. As you inhale and move forward you are working the wrists and shoulders, as you exhale and sit back you are stretching the lower spine.

Take some wide circles with the pelvis in one direction then the other. This will keep the pelvis and hip joints mobile.

Walk your hands to the side of your mat on All Fours to stretch the side of the spine and rib cage.

Alternate Arm and Leg Raises are a good way to work the arms, legs and buttocks and improve general stamina. You should always ensure that you hug your bump in and avoid dipping the lower back. A good way to practice hugging your bump in is to engage the transverse abdominal muscles as you pull the navel in towards the spine. This is a good postural pelvic habit to form early in pregnancy.

Finally you may take one arm up to the ceiling to open up in a wide shoulder rotation. Take a moment to feel the space in the open chest, a liberating move.

I particularly recommend and enjoy the Dynamic Flow Sequence on All Fours, an energising, warming and strengthening sequence which can be practiced all the way through pregnancy.

All Fours postures are part of the safest practices you can choose during your pregnancy.

Standing Postures

Standing postures generally help build strength and stamina in the arms and legs which will support and strengthen the lower back. They can be practiced from trimester II onwards, with variations using supports such as a wall or chair in late pregnancy (34 weeks and over).

Few restrictions apply but:

- if you suffer from high blood pressure, always keep your arms lower than your heart.

- if you suffer from SPD, keep a narrow stance with your knees below your hips or hardly wider.

The Mountain Pose – standing straight with the feet hip width apart - and its variations with feet on the ground can be performed at the beginning of your Yoga practice. It helps with general alignment and neutral holding of the pelvis, a good postural habit to form to support the lower back.

Variations with the arms over the head and out to the side as well as arm rotations constitute a good morning warm up and benefits both arms and stamina. This Yoga practice aims at enhancing the meditative feeling of alertness and relaxation that is often missing in complex Yoga practices mainly because the physical element of the postures distracts you from the Meditation and Breathing practice.

From the Mountain Pose, you can practice the Chair – from standing, bend the knees, sitting back as if sitting on an imaginary chair - with hands on the hips if you need more support or hands over the head for the full posture. This is a strong practice that benefits the thighs and buttocks, therefore ideal if you are planning an active birth. It will also help build strength in the muscles surrounding the pelvis, therefore helping to support the lower back as your bump grows bigger.

Practicing Chair Pose in a dynamic manner or practicing arms movement in a Low Squat position (Horse Stance) can constitute a great warm up or stand alone practice. In addition Wide Pelvic postures such as Low Squats are a great practice in preparation for labour all the way through your pregnancy to keep the pelvis mobile, flexible and open.

However from 34 - 36 weeks, it is best to avoid deep squats and use a chair for support, this will avoid putting too much pressure on the pelvic floor and the cervix.

Some restrictions apply if you are suffering from pelvic pain, Symphysis Pubis Dysfunction (SPD), weakened cervix or low placenta. Take extra care by keeping your feet and legs parallel and hip width apart if you want to practice these positions (always ask your doctor if in doubt).

The Warrior postures – standing with legs wide - build strength and stamina in your legs and arms to improve your general fitness and protect your back. They also help improve your breathing pattern and power of concentration as well as help stretch the side of the body and provide some space for the abdominal organs.

Finally the Sun Salutations or the Moon Salutations are a wonderful dynamic series of poses that can be practiced in trimester II or trimester III as a stand-alone practice. If you only have a few minutes, you could just practice a few rounds of Sun or Moon Salutations to the pace of your breath. This practice will move all of the muscles and joints of the body while leaving you energized.

The postures in Chapter II have been arranged in sequences suitable for either trimester II and trimester III or late pregnancy.

Final Floor Postures

Always take a moment to calm yourself down after a standing sequence and before the Relaxation time. Come to the floor and sit on your mat or a block to practice some Leg Stretches using a Yoga belt, scarf or long sock.

The Leg Stretches in an upright position will be beneficial if you suffer from leg cramps and leverage against the belt helps create some space between the vertebrae.

It is also a good time to practice Pelvis Tilts which will stretch the lower back and also help you become more familiar with the pelvis anatomy.

Finally, an easy Forward Bend will help quieten the mind prior to the Relaxation: you can simply let your head relax forward either sitting cross-legged or in a wide diamond position with the soles of the feet together.

Summary: What Postures to Practice

- Seated Postures will help you gently warm up, keep the spine flexible with open upper back twists, stretch the back of the legs, the side of the rib cage to provide space, the shoulders to counter the effect of postural habits and stimulate the lymphatic system around the breast tissue ahead of breastfeeding. It will also help you connect with the breath, yourself and your baby during Meditation practice.

- All Fours postures are an excellent preparation for labour, help your baby turn to its optimal foetal position around 30-32 weeks, strengthen your wrists and shoulders, stretch the back and provide space for your abdominal organs.

- Standing postures will build strength and stamina in the arms and legs, strengthen the lower back, energise you with the flow of your breath when practiced dynamically, strengthen the back of the legs and stretch the body laterally providing space for the abdominal organs and your baby (from trimester II only to avoid exertion).

- Final Floor postures will help you relax ahead of the final Relaxation, stretch the lower back, become familiar with your pelvis anatomy and stretch the back of the legs to help prevent legs cramps. The effect of all gentle Forward Bends is also calming on the mind.

For demonstration of all sequences by Laurence see her on-line classes at www.pregnancyyogaclasses.com/book

Pelvic Floor Health

It is possible to experience a gentler birth with minimum intervention. For this, preparation is required and pelvic floor exercises are so important towards this goal.

The pelvic floor is a fan shaped multi-layered muscle that supports all of our abdominal organs against gravity. In women, the muscle structure is built around the anal sphincter, urethra and vagina. The structure is wider and more fragmented than in men, therefore also physiologically weaker than in men.

This part of the body is normally taken for granted and we have little awareness of its anatomy and complexity. We associate its functions with our elimination process i.e. a very fundamental and automated bodily process. We only exercise our control over it when having to suppress a natural urge at an inconvenient time and place.

However developing pelvic floor awareness is paramount to a shorter and gentler labour with much reduced chance of tearing. Along with getting your body fit for labour and practicing the Breathing Exercises to help control your mind and pace your stamina, this is the one most important exercise for a healthy delivery.

There are amazing birth stories that demonstrate how being able to consciously relax the pelvic floor resulted in shorter first stage labour and amazingly quick second stage with no tearing. With more body awareness of the pelvic floor and perineum will come a better understanding of how the sphincter works and perhaps more awareness of the sensations in the vagina all the way to the opening of the cervix.

Birth Story from Midwife Gemma

'Sophie B. delivered her first baby very quickly. She arrived at the Maternity Ward at 7pm, quite relaxed and able to bear up really well during her contractions.

She said that thanks to her Yoga practice, she was able to feel what was happening in her body and was able to make sense of her contractions.

During the last push, she used Breathing techniques to help control the release of the baby head slowly which meant she did not need an episiotomy and did not tear at all.'

During the birth, with more tactile sensations, you will be able to feel the baby make its way down the birth canal and control the last push slowly while the baby is gently pushed out and released millimeter by millimeter. You will be aware of the muscle stretching without tearing.

During labour the baby descends down the birth canal and the pressure of the head against the pelvic floor will be all the more effective when the muscle is toned and hence more responsive.

In addition, as you develop your awareness of this part of the body - generally taken for granted up to now - you are becoming able to purposely release, relax and loosen this muscle using your breathing on the exhalation.

You need to learn to contract the pelvic floor so that you are able to relax it. Most exercises include contraction and release. Ideally you should train the body to release on the exhalation, which is what naturally occurs during breathing: the abdominal diaphragm relaxes back up towards the rib cage and the pelvic floor diaphragm domes back in towards the body. As you inhale the abdominal diaphragm extends towards the floor and so does the pelvic floor diaphragm.

Pelvic floor exercises can be practiced on all fours, sitting up or standing. As the aim is to practice 50 -100 contractions/releases per day, it makes sense to take advantage of times when you are sitting in transport or standing in a queue.

This is also the one exercise that you can resume immediately after birth to encourage blood flow to the area and promote healing while regaining control and tone of the muscles.

Pelvic Floor Exercises to Practice

Most practices require you to imagine that the pelvic floor is a three-storey lift and to gradually squeeze to the top foor then release in one go; or squeeze to top floor and gradually release to previous floors. It is good to hold in full squeeze for three seconds prior to releasing.

In order to execute the pelvic floor exercises try the following:

- Place the elbows underneath the shoulders and knees below the hips. Keep the knees wide and let the head completely relax. Support the lower back.

- First Exercise: gradually squeeze to third floor and release in one go. Repeat 10 times.

- Second Exercise: Squeeze all the way to third floor and gradually release to ground. Repeat 10 times.

- Final Exercise: Quick squeeze and release all the way. Repeat 5-8 times initially and progressively build to 10-15. Repeat 3 times.

The above exercises with 50 contractions/releases take less than 10 minutes and should be practiced daily for best results.

You may also want to try to develop your subtle awareness of this part of the body during your Meditation, as you take your attention inwards observing your breath. Pay attention to the movement of the body: the chest, the rib cage, the diaphragm, the abdomen and the pelvic floor. You will become aware of the subtle movement of your pelvic floor up and down while you breathe further increasing your ability to feel sensations.

Summary: Improved Pelvic Floor Muscles Help

- Support the extra weight that you are likely to experience during pregnancy

- Make your baby's descent in the birth canal easier because the pelvic floor is toned and therefore more responsive during first stage labour

- Shorten and ease the second stage labour by allowing release and relax at will during labour

- Healing the perineum after you have given birth to your baby by increasing the circulation of blood into this region

- Toning and regaining control of the pelvic floor in postnatal care

Laurence guides you through the Pelvic Floor Exercises during each of her on-line classes at www.pregnancyyogaclasses.com/book (Menu Pelvic Floor Introduction and Pelvic Floor Exercises)

Yoga for Labour: Labour Positions and Mental Preparation

Giving birth to your baby is not only a very physical experience; it is also a mental challenge and an emotional upheaval.

Physical preparation is certainly essential but mental preparation is key.

Being mentally prepared will help support you on a physical level, avoiding exhaustion, meaning that you will be in good emotional shape to welcome your baby to the world.

Understanding the role of the brain and hormones during labour is critical so that we can use Breathing techniques and Relaxation to train and practice ahead of labour. With adequate preparation it is possible to have the natural birth that you wish with minimum medical intervention and drugs. What could be better for you and your baby?

Active Birth Principle

The concept of active birth is not new to the world and active birthing has been practiced over the centuries in many parts of the world. In the case of an active birth, you will have sole control over your body and total ability to live the experience fully without medical intervention. Drugs could have adverse effects on the health of your baby. You can move and change position with ease, you are fully aware throughout your baby's birth.

This is just the reverse of an actively managed birth when the complete power of control is taken away from you. In this case, you are nothing but a passive patient under somebody else's control.

The evolution of childbirth practices in recent times is interesting. It is only in the fifties that medical intervention started becoming more present. It was indeed in support of women empowerment against traditional views that anaesthetics were offered to women, initially in the form of chloroform. Birthing generally occurred with the mother completely unconscious.

Over the last decades the types of available anaesthetics have increased and the choice of drugs now gives women maximum awareness, more mobility and somewhat more control during the birthing process while protecting the safety of the baby. Unfortunately, the emergency Caesarian sections rate is very high, leaving the normal delivery rate in the UK in 2009 at only 46%.

Active Birthing Positions

Imagine the pelvis as two bowls, a larger bowl with the upper rim connected to the abdomen and the lower rim connected to a smaller bowl.

You can feel the upper rim of your pelvis by pressing your hands over the two large bones just below the waist. Follow the Iliac Crest down the front to the Anterior Superior Iliac Spine (ASIS) or Hip Points and to the back to the Posterior Superior Iliac Spine (PSIS), two nobly points located about an inch either side of the spine.

Now the lower part of the smaller bowl is the actual doorway to the world for your baby. Move your hands from your sit bones forward to the pubic bone and back to the coccyx forming a diamond shape where the pelvic floor or pelvic diaphragm sits.

Active birthing with upright positions during labour can help maximize the pelvic space for your baby. For the second stage, if you are able to lean forward to a wall or bedhead or be supported by your partner squatting between their knees, the sacrum and coccyx will flare out and you will offer more space for your baby. Conversely, the traditional position on your back with legs up will have the sacrum and coccyx moving towards your baby's space potentially reducing it by 25-30%.

There are also many optimal labour positions I can recommend during the earlier parts of labour and first stage to encourage the cervix to dilate.

Standing positions include Hip Rolls against the wall or taking large steps walks. You may also practice Hip Rolls supported on a birthing ball or a chair. Alternatively other active birthing positions may be on All Fours or kneeling.

It is important to practice a wide range of positions so that you can see what works best during labour and feel that you have some options with which to work.

All positions aim to bring blood flow to the cervix while putting you in a wide pelvic position to facilitate the dilation process and the transition i.e. your baby's descent into the birth canal. All positions take advantage of the downward force of gravity.

In addition these postures allow you to keep your attention inwards either looking to the wall or the floor, keeping your attention focused on your Breathing techniques with minimum light.

The Role of Hormones During Labour

During labour the hormone that prompts contractions is called oxytocin. This hormone is regulated by the hypothalamus, the part of our ancestral primal brain responsible for our mammalian instincts. The oxytocin release kicks in when your baby is ready for birth. This effectively triggers contractions and is the onset of labour.

Unfortunately the release of oxytocin is constrained by adrenaline release which is regulated by our neo cortex, our rational controlling brain. Any anxiety, fear, tension or anger will increase our adrenaline release which will slow down the oxytocin release and in turn slow down contractions and labour. In addition adrenaline and fear will make the contractions less effective and more painful as the whole body tenses up.

In order to let the body do its work it is important to practice moving inwards through the use of Relaxation, Breathing and Meditation.

Realising that the body knows what to do and that what is happening to you during labour is what is meant to happen can help build confidence in your body, suppress any sensation of panic and, whilst retaining some control, help you surrender to the natural and powerful process of labour.

Oxytocin release will be stimulated by your calm Breathing techniques, calming the mind, keeping within the moment, keeping to yourself, remaining warm and in a dark and quiet environment.

You can practice Breathing techniques and Visualisation exercises in wide pelvic positions during that time to keep the body moving in line with the principles of the active birth.

Training your partner ahead of time can be very helpful. They will be able to guide you through the next Breathing exercise or posture while understanding that minimum interaction with your mind is best for you and your baby to keep good progress.

Summary: How Yoga Can Help You Have The Natural Birth You Wish

- It is possible to have the natural birth you wish for: prepare physically and mentally.

- Physical Preparation: understanding the impact of positions on labour and your baby is critical. Yoga helps prepare with active birthing positions using the downward force of gravity and maximizing pelvic space.

- Mental Preparation: the role of the brain and the role of hormones in labour are such that Yogic Breathing and Meditation become a critical tool during labour.

Laurence talks about the Physiology of Birth as part of each of her on-line classes and the special bonus class Labour Preparation. See www.pregnancyyogaclasses.com/book

Yogic Breathing: Conscious Breathing

Yogic Breathing as well as Energy Control techniques contribute to maintaining the health of an expectant mum. At the time of pregnancy, maintaining a sound and good breathing pattern is of utmost importance. Just like your unborn child gets nutrients from your food it also gets oxygen from the air you inhale. Above all a good breathing pattern ensures an improved life force to your baby.

In addition Conscious Breathing is an essential preparation for labour. Prenatal care in many parts of the world include Breathing practice specifically for Labour.

Regular practice of the following Yoga Breathing techniques will maximize your ability to manage your labour in line with the principles of active birthing.

Conscious Breathing techniques help in releasing emotional tension at the time of labour. Focusing the mind on the breath and on specific parts of the body while breathing will simultaneously focus and distract the mind.

You will feel calmer, less subject to anxiety which will maximize the release of oxytocin, minimize the release of adrenaline and therefore help make contractions more effective and less painful.

During the first stage of labour it is essential to avoid the surge of adrenaline that comes with fear and anxiety. When adrenaline is released into the body the muscles prepare for a fight or flight response, sending all the blood to the limbs and depriving the uterus from the blood flow it needs to progress the transition and contractions. This makes the contractions less effective and more painful.

With preparation, using Breathing and Visualisation techniques you will be able to eliminate the physical reactions that hinder the birthing process. Thus each contraction will be more effective and their number will be less if the process is quicker.

Breathing will also help you to surrender to the power of nature while providing you with a haven of peace between contractions, a much needed space to recuperate, save your energy and pace yourself.

Traditionally, the so-called 'Pranayama' practice in Sanskrit is ideally performed at dawn or dusk before Meditation and before or after the Asana practice (practice of Yoga postures). However you may practice Conscious Breathing at any time, whether you have set some time aside first thing in the morning or last thing prior to going to bed. You may also take advantage of the time on a public transport journey.

Breathing Exercises to Practice

Use the following exercises at the beginning of each Yoga practice for just a few minutes. Regular practice will help condition the mind and body so that you can achieve a peaceful state at will.

Firstly sit in a comfortable position, preferably cross-legged on the floor, perhaps using a rolled blanket or cushion to elevate the pelvis and ensure that the spine is lifted through the back of the body to allow the energy to move freely up and down the spine.

Close your eyes and start by dedicating this time to your practice. Consciously leave aside any tension and excitement of the day, any material concerns and start by drawing your attention inwards, observing your breathing pattern. Notice the flow of the breath, its pace and quality and refrain from judging or interfering. Any distraction or thoughts that come into the mind simply return to observing your breathing once you have acknowledged the thought. Then continue to observe the air passing in and out of the nostrils, notice the cool air as you breathe in and the warmer air as you breathe out.

Finally observe the movement of the body as you breathe, notice the movement of the chest, the rib-cage, the diaphragm and the abdomen. Can you feel the movement of the pelvic floor or pelvic diaphragm in tune with the abdominal diaphragm?

- Start counting to four on the inhale and counting to four on the exhale. During this exercise you are aiming to lengthen the exhale to double the length of the inhale. This is to release mental, physical and emotional tension. Never let yourself be out of breath and never hold the breath during the exercise. All your breathing should be through the nose. Progressively build the count of the exhale to 8 while the count of the inhale remains at four. Once you reach a 4 to 8 ratio, or perhaps 3 to 6 if this is more comfortable for you, repeat for another 6-8 rounds then return to normal breathing.

- Take your attention to your sit bones and the contact of the floor, visualise the earth beneath you. As you inhale imagine you are breathing in the earth energy through the front of the body and over the crown of the head. As you exhale visualise the energy cascading down the back of the body and down into the earth. Repeat for a few rounds for a calming and grounding meditative practice. Become familiar with this wave, like the motion of the breath.

Breathing Exercises for Labour to Practice

The following techniques are employed during the first stage of labour and during crowning of your baby's head. Try them out and decide which may work for you. Remember that some may work better for you than others, therefore practice each so you can use your choice on the big day. It is a good idea to practice with your birth partner so they can guide you by performing the exercise near you and lead you into it.

- Take slow deep breaths into the abdomen at the end of each contraction. When you exhale, make sure to release all tension. This will help you and your baby recuperate between contractions, conserving energy and stamina.

- Focus all your attention on observing and relaxing some other part of your body each time a contraction rises. This can help you dissociate from overwhelming sensations.

- Try focusing on the air passing in and out of the nostrils to distract the mind from the contractions.

- Focus on the energy breath. Inhale through the front of the body, exhale through the back and focus on the exhalation only. This will help take the attention to the back and reduce the overwhelming sensations at the front where the contractions are often felt.

The following two exercises are particularly helpful to help you refrain from pushing as your baby's head crowns.

- Breathe in slowly through your nose and breathe out through your mouth. Keep the lips slightly parted, imagine that you are blowing a feather through a tiny gap without pursing the lips to keep the mouth completely relaxed. This is an important factor in helping to let go of tension on the pelvic floor.

- Alternatively repeat the above and try producing a light humming sound on the exhalation.

Summary: Conscious Breathing Techniques Help

- Calm and focus the mind during contractions

- Keep fear and adrenaline at bay

- Provide recuperation between contractions

- Surrender while providing you with more control and less anxiety

- Release emotional tension at the time of labour

All techniques are demonstrated and recorded by Laurence as part of her on-line classes at www.pregnancyyogaclasses.com/book (Menu Breathing Exercises, Meditation and special bonus class Labour Preparation)

Relaxation and Visualisation

Relaxation at the end of a Yoga practice is essential to reap the benefits of the practice. This is providing time for the muscles to heal, recuperate and strengthen, for the mind to be quietened and appeased and on the emotional side for you to be satisfied that you are setting some time for yourself to nurture yourself and rest. Remember that by nurturing yourself and reflecting on the feeling of calm, love and quiet, you are also nurturing your baby and stimulating the hormones that will make you and your baby feel good.

You should set aside 10-20 minutes everyday for a quiet Meditation or rest. Up to late pregnancy you may lie on your side or at any time during the pregnancy you can prop yourself up to a 45 degree angle using bolsters or stacked up pillows and rolled blankets.

Once you have established and conditioned your body and mind for Relaxation, you will be able to access this safe and special space beyond the mat and during your everyday life, providing you with a haven of peace and quiet whatever stressful conditions you may find yourself in. It will also give you more control over yourself and enhance the quality of life around you.

You will think clearer, improve your power of concentration and help yourself feel happier, calmer and more energised.

During pregnancy it may also lower your discomfort level, improving the efficiency of your body by lowering blood pressure level, heart rate, muscle tension and breathing rate and provide sound sleep.

Here is how you can get started, perhaps setting a clock for 15 minutes

- Keep aside a routine time for relaxing, preferably when you are not too sleepy. However if you fall asleep then that is fine as well.

- Select a quiet place and prop yourself up.

- Wear comfortable loose clothing and a blanket to keep you warm.

- Set a timer.

- You can use Silent Meditation techniques or use the Relaxation and Visualisations included in Chapter III.

Start by taking your attention inwards and take this opportunity to practice one of the Breathing Exercises provided. Notice your breath, notice your body move with the breath. Start counting your inhale and exhale to four, repeating for a few rounds.

You can then use techniques such as Yoga Nidra, a technique that consists of taking attention to all the parts of the body from toes to head, with the view to mentally release and relax each body part. Remain silent for a few more minutes clearing your mind of any thoughts for a deep Relaxation.

Alternatively pre-record Visualisation texts such as the ones included in Chapter III and play them back.

Pregnancy specific Visualisations aim to build confidence that your body will know how to deliver your baby as well as it knew how to conceive and bring it safely to term. Your mind needs to surrender to the force of nature and paradoxically this is what gives you more control of yourself and your birth.

Other pregnancy Visualisations aim to enhance the emotional bond with your baby.

Labour specific Visualisations can help condition the mind and the body as you are practicing and preparing for the birth. They specifically help you to imagine how you will be reacting to the contractions and how to breathe through them.

Birth Visualisation Exercises to Practice

First ensure that you are seated comfortably and proceed with your usual Relaxation technique, focusing on the breath then scanning all the parts of the body. Once you are totally relaxed you can try the following texts pre-recorded with your voice. While recording, read calmly taking care to include many pauses where the text is marked by several dots.

- The following Visualisation helps to recuperate between contractions so that you preserve your energy and dissociate yourself from overwhelming contractions.

  The contraction just subsided..... breathe deeply..... inhale and let the air fill your tummy..... gently massaging your baby..... let your baby know that you are taking a break together..... exhale and release any tension..... As you inhale and exhale, let the motion gently soothe you and your baby..... welcome this peace between contractions..... you are recuperating..... preserving your energy for your next contraction and your baby's arrival.

- This Visualisation helps to stimulate baby's descent in the birth canal.

  Feel the wave of energy moving up on the inhale and down the back of the body on the exhale..... With each exhale..... imagine your baby is moving down..... you are pushing with your mind..... Now feel the strength, the irresistible force of a contraction..... surrender to its intensity..... now with each exhale..... imagine your baby moving down..... making the contraction all the more effective.

Work on these exercises at the end of a Relaxation or Meditation to help condition your body and mind for the birth.

Summary: Relaxation, Meditation and Visualisation Practice Are Essential for

- Learning to connect with yourself

- Calming your mind

- Increasing focus and clarity of mind

- Promoting self healing and rest

- Emotional bonding with your baby

- Conditioning for labour

Yoga for Emotional Preparation: Bond Now With Your Baby

Babies Have Emotional Needs in Utero

Pregnancy is the time when you share a true bond with your baby. Experiencing for the first time your baby move inside you is truly magical and as the baby grows there are physical and emotional interactions that take place to which your baby is receptive.

Birth isn't the beginning; in fact it is a continuation of another phase of life; the life of your unborn child in your womb. Your baby already becomes a family member from the first few weeks of its development in your womb and for first babies it creates the family.

Undoubtedly to an extent unborn babies also have emotional needs. They too need to be nurtured and loved, accepted and acknowledged. And this is where prenatal bonding steps in. Prenatal bonding with your unborn baby prepares you for bonding with your baby once born and makes the reality of carrying your baby more present.

During the last few months of pregnancy you are likely to find a heel that ripples across your abdomen. The father can push mildly to find a shoulder or foot and he will find the baby pushing back. Your baby will recognize its father's touch and speech. Finding your baby responding to your touch is indeed a thrilling experience.

Music is pre-linguistic and helps in establishing language skills for your baby. Listening to music can provide healthy stimulation for the development of the child.

Yoga sound vibrations in particular for instance AUM chanting can also create a reassuring sound and vibration that your baby will recognize after birth. This is a practice I particularly enjoyed during the end of my pregnancy and I really felt my baby was receptive to the sounds and vibration. Later on this helped me calm my baby prior to going to sleep.

For many months after her birth I also used the meditative Ujjayi Victorious breath. This is when you lengthen the breathing, restricting the space at the back of the throat to produce a hissing sound. 10 to 20 rounds worked wonders to calm our baby at nap time.

Communicate with Your Baby

An ideal way of communication between a mother and unborn child is by Relaxation and touch. By massaging your tummy and focusing on love, hormones get released which help you relax and help soften your tummy and in turn may calm your baby.

It is important to feel relaxed at the time of your pregnancy, hence devote some time for yourself. This will make your baby feel that it is safe and secure within.

Conversely it has been established that babies are able to pick up on tension and stress and are affected by high levels of adrenaline and cortisol present in the mother's body. Medical studies show that high executives under a lot of pressure can have similar effects experienced by drug addicts and have smaller babies.

Meditation Exercises for Bonding to Practice

Try this Meditation for bonding with your baby by drawing the attention inwards to intentionally connect with it.

- At a time when you are not sleepy sit up supported with some cushions against a wall.

- Take one hand to your heart centre and place the other hand on your baby. Focus your attention to your breath and then focus on your heart. Experience feelings of love and happiness. Expand these feelings and visualise a transfer from your heart into your bump, from one hand to your other hand. Visualise the sharing of this feeling which is triggering a feel-good energy in you, positively affecting your emotional health and hence your and in turn your baby's physical health.

Heart Centre Meditation is one of the most natural yet effective practices. The heart is an incredible organ, not only the cardiac muscle that supports our life system but also a gland emitting hormones. It is also the seat of about 40,000 neurons (normally located in the brain) that allow the heart to communicate with the brain and other parts of the body in many ways: neurologically (through transmissions of nerve impulses), biochemically (through hormones and synapses), biophysically (through waves) and also energetically (through electromagnetic field interactions).

Hence, the heart communicates to the brain and body sending messages of emotional and intuitive quality. Because of recent medical findings in this field the heart can be called the emotional and intelligent force behind what we call our gut feeling or intuition.

By stimulating your feeling of love you are nurturing yourself and ensuring that your baby also feels nurtured and loved.

Prepare for After the Birth

During pregnancy we are so engrossed with preparing for the birth, reading pregnancy books, attending prenatal appointments etc., that strangely the journey (from trimester I moving to trimester II and trimester III) seems to end with the final step i.e the birth or the end goal, without consideration for the ongoing needs of ourselves and our baby. It can become a process.

Although we do prepare our baby's clothes, bedding, bedroom, cot, furniture, wall paper etc... we spend little time focusing on our baby's actual needs after the birth. This is because this belongs to another stage of life somehow and we find difficulty in imagining it until we face its reality.

Parenthood preparation, whether attending a class or reading books, can help prepare you with realistic expectations of you as a parent and of your baby. It can be confidence building and help you feel up to the task, bring a positive image of your adequacy as a new mother and parent and assure you that you are doing everything to take care of your baby. It will help you be more relaxed around your baby and around others.

Your baby's needs are very simple and can be divided between sleep, activity and feed. Activity largely includes development, interactions, walks, changing and bathing. It can be disheartening for parents to see their babies cry and feel that they have no ways to pacify them. It is helpful to recognize that babies at that time have no other way of expressing themselves and this is part of their emotional communication.

Parents are encouraged to trust their instincts and within a few weeks of getting to know your baby, it will become easier to pick up on its needs and the various sounds it uses to communicate. You can however feel lost between the different schools of thought be it the on-demand feeding or the routine feeding regime and this contradictory advice may not help you find your natural instincts.

Phillip and I found understanding and translating our baby's needs in terms of the cycle of sleep, feed and activity an invaluable help. When the order of the cycle is repeated over and over, any change of mood in your baby, any slight fidgeting means that it is ready for the next phase. It is only a matter of picking up on it early enough so that your baby does not get irritated… (our reference on this topic was the Baby Whisperer from Tracy Hogg).

This is a wonderful time, enjoy every minute of it.

Summary: Connecting with Your Baby on an Emotional Level

- Touch your baby through your tummy and play

- Send a message of love to your baby during Meditation

- Practice guided Relaxation and Meditation

- Chant sounds and songs

- Prepare for after the birth: understanding your baby's emotional needs

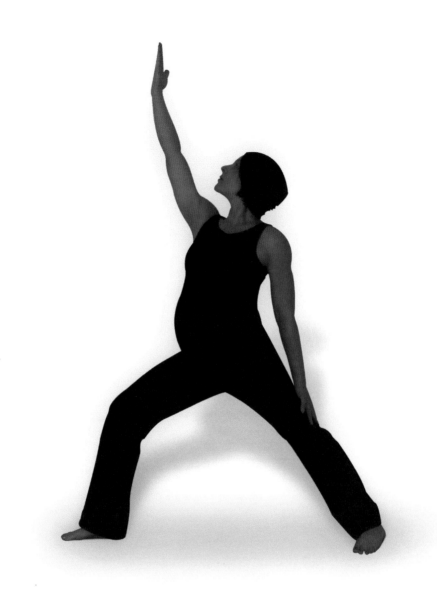

Chapter II

Yoga Sequences to Practice

This section will help you build a home practice. You can choose sequences from the sub sections based on how you feel like practicing at each time of the day, the time available and what your body needs.

For your convenience the full instructions are on the left page with the corresponding pictures on the right page. The numbers correspond to key postures in the sequence with easy reference on the picture page. Once you are familiar with the full instructions, as a quick guide, you can use the picture page only following the titles below the pictures.

Yoga Sequences to Practice: Overview

You will find the sequences in the following order:

Gentle Seated Warm Up Sequence: The 4 sequences from which to choose offer gentle warm up to your practice, focusing on gently moving the shoulder joints, stretching the legs and warming the spine.

All Fours Sequences: These 4 sequences are ideal as a warm up to a longer practice or, if time is short, as a quick stand alone work out in the morning. Choose one or two sequences at a time. The sequences focus on strengthening the wrists and shoulders, warming the spine, stretching the lower back, building stamina and opening the sides of the ribcage and the hips.

Standing Sequences for Trimester II and Trimester III. These are 4 sequences to practice singly or a combination of 2 repeated twice on each side. Standing sequences are great to build strength and stamina in the legs and arms, strengthen the lower back and bring energy to the body.

More specifically:

   - *Sun Salutations:* This dynamic sequence to the flow of the breath will help warm all the joints in the body; an energising sequence.

- *Warrior Sequence:* This helps build strong arms and legs and helps you feel emotionally stable, secure and confident.

- *Squat Sequence:* These exercises are for use singly or in combination. Each exercise can be repeated 4 times, dynamically holding the squat position for one breath (i.e. one inhalation and one exhalation). These postures are great for the legs and stamina and can be used in combination with any sequences for warm up and strength building.

- *Moon Salutations:* Here is a more gentle and meditative dynamic sequence to gently stretch the legs, chest and hips. This sequence is traditionally practiced at dawn for its calming effect.

Standing Sequences for Late Pregnancy: Most of the above sequences can be practiced in late pregnancy. In this section they have been adapted to include the use of a chair or stool which will help ensure that you do not overwork or send too much weight down the cervix. Avoid low squats without support from 34-36 weeks.

Final Floor Sequences: Use one of the 3 sequences to finish your practice and wind yourself down prior to the Relaxation. You may also use these sequences as a stand-alone 10 minute practice in the evening to stretch the legs and prevent leg cramps.

How to Practice

Always start with a Breathing exercise seated cross-legged for 8-10 breaths then move on to your practice and finish with a Breathing exercise either sitting up or lying on your left side (Short Lying Relaxation) for 5 mins. If time permits a full Relaxation is preferable (10mins +). In trimester I build your practice from the Warming or Calming routines only. In later trimesters, if you are practicing several sequences, choose one sequence of each section in the above order or any of the routines suggested.

Sequence Builder Guide

Use the following guide to build your home practice routine. Decide first for how long you want to practice and which sequence is applicable according to the time of day or type of routine you need. This will help you navigate down the first column to select a row of sequences.

Build your home practice routine from the exercises detailed in the next section, not forgetting Breathing and Relaxation practice before and after the postures sequences.

Time/Type	Before	Postures	Postures	Postures	Postures	Finish
AM 20 mins Warming	Breathing Exercise	Seated Sequence	All Fours Sequence			Breathing Exercise
AM 25 mins Energising	Breathing Exercise	All Fours Sequence	Standing Sequence	Final Floor Sequence		Short Lying Relaxation
Day 50mins Complete	Breathing Exercise	All Fours Sequence	2 x Standing Sequences	Final Floor Sequence		Full Relaxation
Day 60mins Complete	Breathing Exercise	Seated Sequence	All Fours Sequence	2 x Standing Sequences	Final Floor Sequence	Full Relaxation
PM 35 mins Energising	Breathing Exercise	Seated Sequence	2x Standing Sequence	Final Floor Sequence		Short Lying Relaxation
PM 25 mins Energising	Breathing Exercise	All Fours Sequence	Standing Sequence	Final Floor Sequence		Breathing Exercise
PM 25 mins Calming	Breathing Exercise	All Fours Sequence	Final Floor Sequence			Full Relaxation
PM 25 mins Calming	Breathing Exercise	Seated Sequence	Final Floor Sequence			Full Relaxation

Instructions and Yoga Sequences

Gentle Seated Warm Up Sequences

These postures can be practiced all the way through your pregnancy. If you are suffering from pelvic pain and in particular Symphysis Pubis Pain keep your knees in front of your hips at all times and avoid taking the knees out wide. For the benefits of these see Chapter I Seated Postures.

For more information or for demonstration of all sequences by Laurence see **www.pregnancyyogaclasses.com/book**

Instructions: Cross-Legged Gentle Warm-up

1. Start in simple cross-legged (Neutral) position.

2. Inhale taking the arms with the palms up out to the sides to above the head, exhale lowering the arms forward and reach the hands to the floor in front.

3. Inhale sliding the finger tips back towards you, leave the left hand touching the front foot and place the right hand behind the right sit bone while reaching through the crown of the head, exhale turning the head and look behind the right shoulder. Feel the stretch through the collar bones.

4. Inhale turning yourself back to centre, exhale placing the right hand to the side of the right hip. Inhale reaching out to the side with the left arm up above the head, exhale Side Bend towards the right. Feel the stretch along the left rib cage.

5. Inhale moving back to Neutral position.

Repeat to the other side and repeat the whole sequence at least once.

Cross-Legged Gentle Warm-up

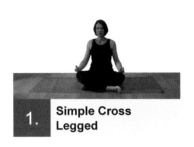

1. **Simple Cross Legged**

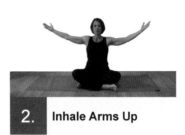

2. **Inhale Arms Up**

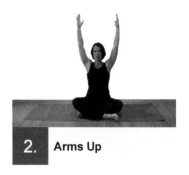

2. **Arms Up**

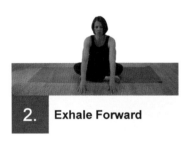

2. **Exhale Forward**

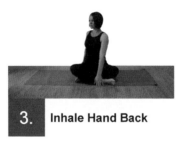

3. **Inhale Hand Back**

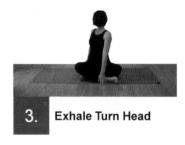

3. **Exhale Turn Head**

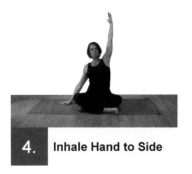

4. **Inhale Hand to Side**

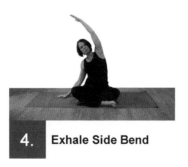

4. **Exhale Side Bend**

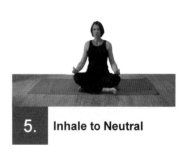

5. **Inhale to Neutral**

Instructions: One Leg Forward Bend Warm-up

1. From simple cross-legged (Neutral) position, open the right leg out to the side with the left foot resting towards the inner right thigh.

2. Turn towards the right leg, sit straight and flex the foot (toes to ceiling). Inhale moving the arms out to the side, exhale reaching the hands forward to the right leg, taking care not to constrain any part of your bump.

3. Inhale moving back towards you, place the right hand to the left foot and the left finger tips behind the left sit bone, exhale turning the head and look behind the left shoulder.

4. Inhale turning the head back to centre and exhale. Lean onto the left hand behind the left sit bone. Inhale lifting the hips up using the leverage of the left knee, take the right arm up and above the head, exhale lowering the body to floor.

5. Slide the back of the right hand inside the right knee. Inhale moving the left arm out to the side and up to the ceiling, pointing to ceiling gaze up to the open left palm, exhale lowering the arm and return to Neutral.

Repeat to the other side and repeat the whole sequence at least once.

One Leg Forward Bend Warm-up

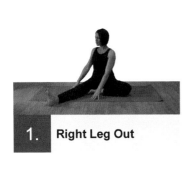

1. Right Leg Out

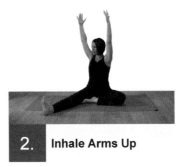

2. Inhale Arms Up

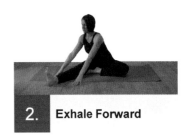

2. Exhale Forward

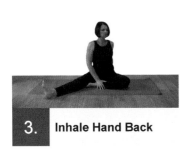

3. Inhale Hand Back

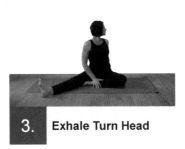

3. Exhale Turn Head

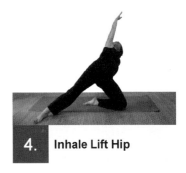

4. Inhale Lift Hip

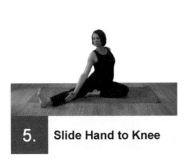

5. Slide Hand to Knee

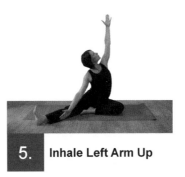

5. Inhale Left Arm Up

Instructions: Hip Opening Sequence

1. From simple cross-legged (Neutral) position bring the soles of the feet together, hold the feet for 4 breaths. (Butterfly Pose). Come back to Neutral and interlace the hands.

2. Inhale raising both arms up above the head, exhale pressing the palms to the ceiling. Stay for 4 breaths. Repeat changing over the interlace of the hands by one finger.

3. Bring the soles of the feet together (Butterfly Pose) and rock gently from side to side to open the hips.

4. Continue with Hip Rolls moving the body around from one side to the other in a circle in each direction, then return to Neutral position.

5. Put the left ankle underneath the right knee and pick up the right leg and place the right ankle over the left knee. Keep the feet flexed. A narrow triangle should be formed with the knees in front of the hips and shins parallel to the edge of the mat in front and one above the other (Fire Log Pose). Hold for 7 breaths and repeat changing sides.

6. Alternative position for 5.

Hip Opening Sequence

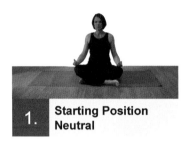

1. Starting Position Neutral

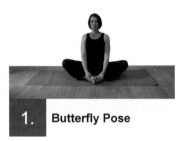

1. Butterfly Pose

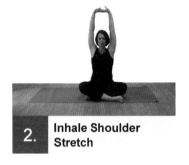

2. Inhale Shoulder Stretch

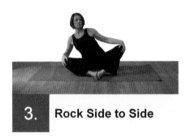

3. Rock Side to Side

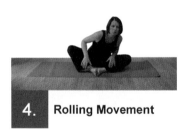

4. Rolling Movement

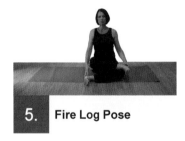

5. Fire Log Pose

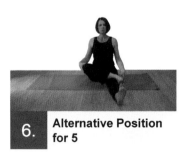

6. Alternative Position for 5

Instructions: Gentle Spine Stretches

1. From simple cross-legged (Neutral) position inhale reaching the arms out to the side and above the head, exhale turning the palms down and lower. Repeat four times.

2. Interlace the hands to the front, inhale lifting the arms up above the head. Stay for 4 breaths and repeat changing over the interlace of the hands by one finger. Release the arms.

3. Place the left hand to the front foot, the right finger tips behind the right sit bone. Inhale reaching up through the crown of the head to your full height, exhale turning the head to look behind the right shoulder. Repeat to the other side.

4. Place the right hand to the side. Inhale stretching the left arm up above the head, exhale Side Bend to the right. Repeat to the other side.

5. Place both feet flat on the floor in front of the hips, place the hands around the knees. Inhale, using the hands for leverage tilt the pelvis forward as you reach upwards expanding your body, exhale tucking the tailbone under and, thinking of stretching the spine, round the spine in a C shape. Repeat 5 times.

6. Bring the soles of the feet together with knees in a wide diamond shape, feet away from you. Slide the hands under the ankles to cup the feet, fold forward gently releasing the head. Concentrate on the breath. Lift up slowly.

Gentle Spine Stretches

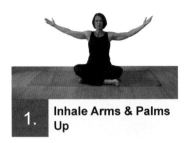

1. Inhale Arms & Palms Up

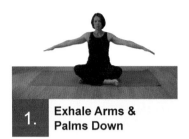

1. Exhale Arms & Palms Down

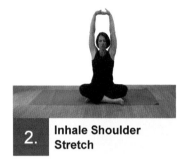

2. Inhale Shoulder Stretch

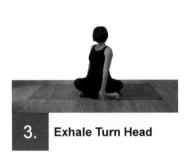

3. Exhale Turn Head

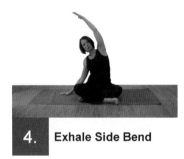

4. Exhale Side Bend

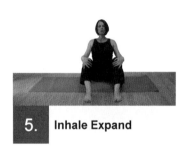

5. Inhale Expand

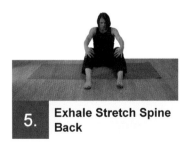

5. Exhale Stretch Spine Back

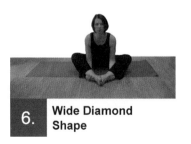

6. Wide Diamond Shape

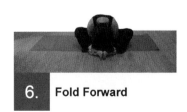

6. Fold Forward

All Fours Sequences

These postures can be practiced all the way through your pregnancy even when suffering from the SPD front pelvic pain in which case you should keep both knees or feet on the floor. For the benefits of these postures see Chapter I All Fours Postures.

Instructions: Cat Variations

1. Start on All Fours (Neutral Cat), setting the hands underneath the shoulders, knees under hips, hip width apart. Hug your bump in to support the back.

2. Inhale leaning forward working the wrists and shoulders, exhale leaning back over the heels stretching the lower back. Repeat 6 times and come back to Neutral.

3. Make large movements with the hips around in one direction then change direction. Repeat 4 times each side and come back to Neutral.

4. Inhale lifting one arm up, exhale lowering the arm taking care to keep a flat back. Change arms and repeat. Carry out the whole exercise twice.

5. Inhale extending one leg back, exhale lowering the leg taking care to keep a flat back. Either lift the foot to hip level keeping the hips square towards the floor or keep the toes on the mat while extending through the heel. Repeat as for the arms.

6. Inhale lifting one arm and the opposite leg, exhale lowering the arm. Change sides and repeat.

Cat Variations

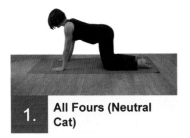

1. All Fours (Neutral Cat)

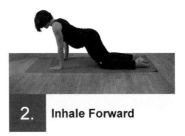

2. Inhale Forward

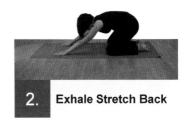

2. Exhale Stretch Back

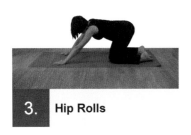

3. Hip Rolls

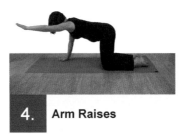

4. Arm Raises

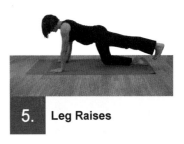

5. Leg Raises

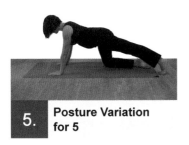

5. Posture Variation for 5

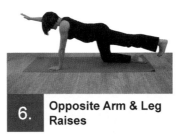

6. Opposite Arm & Leg Raises

Instructions: Dynamic Flow

1. Start on All Fours (Neutral Cat). Inhale and on the exhale, firming hands and knees against the floor and releasing the head, round the back and stretch the spine to the ceiling (Cat Stretch).

2. Inhale coming back to Neutral Cat, tuck the toes under, exhale lifting the tailbone up to the ceiling (Down Dog). Press the weight back and straighten the legs.

3. Inhale releasing the knees to the floor, exhale sitting back on the heels and keeping the hands on the mat stretch the spine and then rest.

4. Inhale coming up to Neutral Cat and repeat from 1-3 four times to the flow of the breath.

5. From Neutral Cat walk the hands to one side feeling the stretch to the waist on the opposite side (Side Cat). Repeat to the other side. Carry out the whole exercise a few times.

6. Sit back and rest for a few breaths in Supported Child's pose.

Dynamic Flow

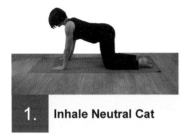

1. Inhale Neutral Cat

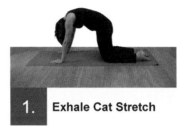

1. Exhale Cat Stretch

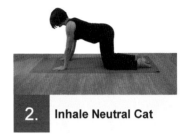

2. Inhale Neutral Cat

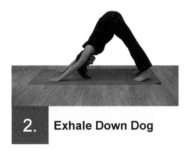

2. Exhale Down Dog

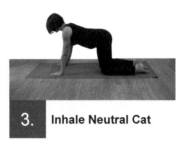

3. Inhale Neutral Cat

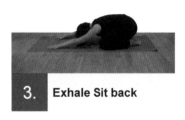

3. Exhale Sit back

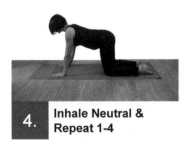

4. Inhale Neutral & Repeat 1-4

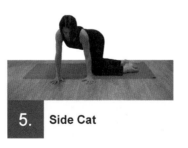

5. Side Cat

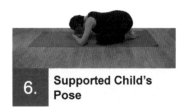

6. Supported Child's Pose

Instructions: Shoulder and Lateral Stretch

1. Start on All Fours (Neutral Cat). Inhale and on the exhale, firming hands and knees against the floor, round the back and stretch the spine to the ceiling. Release the head (Cat Stretch). Repeat 5 times.

2. Place the right foot forward outside the right hand to allow room for your bump. Inhale raising arms up and above the head, exhale tucking the tailbone under. Inhale and on the next exhale release the arms.

3. Ideally tuck the toes of the left foot under and straighten the leg extending through the left heel. Alternatively stay in same position. Lean onto the left hand, lifting the right arm up hand to the ceiling, stretch through the chest in a shoulder rotation.

4. Come back to Neutral Cat and repeat 2 and 3 for the other side (left foot forward).

5. From Neutral Cat put your weight onto the right hand and right knee whilst extending your left leg out, resting the left foot flat on the floor parallel to the short side of the mat. Inhale lifting the hips while pressing on the right knee and extend the left arm up to the ceiling (Side Plank). Stay for one breath. Repeat to the other side.

6. From Neutral Cat slide the right arm underneath the body to the left hand (Thread the Needle). If your bump allows rest the side of your head and shoulder on the floor. Stay for 2 breaths, sending the breath to the space between the shoulder blades. Inhale and return to Neutral Cat. Repeat for the other side.

7. Rest the elbows, under shoulders, and lower arms onto the mat. Keeping a flat back extend the right arm forward while stretching the tailbone back. Feel the stretch to the rib cage and arm pit. Repeat for the other side.

Shoulder and Lateral Stretch

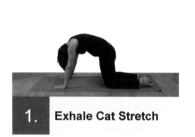

1. **Exhale Cat Stretch**

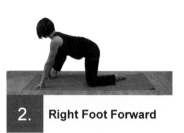

2. **Right Foot Forward**

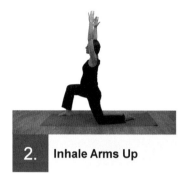

2. **Inhale Arms Up**

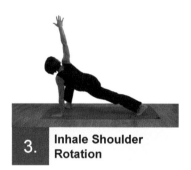

3. **Inhale Shoulder Rotation**

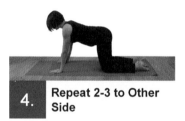

4. **Repeat 2-3 to Other Side**

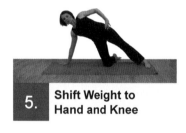

5. **Shift Weight to Hand and Knee**

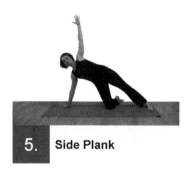

5. **Side Plank**

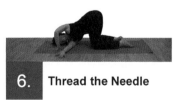

6. **Thread the Needle**

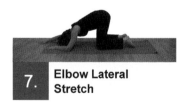

7. **Elbow Lateral Stretch**

Instructions: Hip Opening Sequence

1. From All Fours (Neutral Cat) make large Hip Roll movements with the hips around in each direction. Repeat 4 times each way and return to Neutral Cat.

2. Lift the right knee and rotate in large or medium circles. Repeat 4 times in both directions. Repeat with the left knee and return to Neutral Cat.

3. Place the right foot forward outside the right hand to allow room for your bump. Inhale raising arms up above the head, exhale tucking the tailbone under. Inhale and on the exhale release the arms. Repeat for the other side.

4. From Neutral Cat lift the right knee and place it one third of the way towards and behind the right wrist. Place the right heel in line with the left wrist and knee. Slide the left leg back directly behind the left hip. Check that the right thigh is parallel to the long side of the mat and the right heel underneath the left hip. Stay or come down to the elbows for 4 breaths (Pigeon Pose). Repeat to the other side.

5. In late pregnancy from 34 weeks, practice with a rolled blanket or a large block underneath the pelvis to support the extra weight and avoid over stretching. Remain supported on the hands.

6. Sit back and rest for a few breaths in Supported Child's Pose.

Hip Opening Sequence

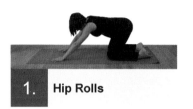

1. Hip Rolls

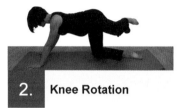

2. Knee Rotation

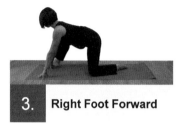

3. Right Foot Forward

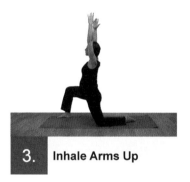

3. Inhale Arms Up

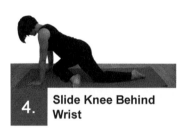

4. Slide Knee Behind Wrist

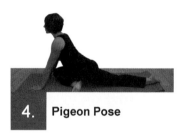

4. Pigeon Pose

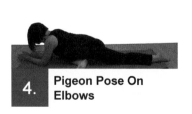

4. Pigeon Pose On Elbows

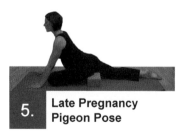

5. Late Pregnancy Pigeon Pose

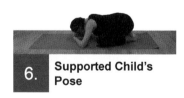

6. Supported Child's Pose

Standing Sequences for Trimester II and III

Standing postures generally help build strength and stamina in the arms and legs which will support and strengthen the lower back. They can be practiced from trimester II onwards, with variations using supports such as a wall or chair in late pregnancy (34 weeks and over).

Few restrictions apply:

If you suffer from high blood pressure, always keep your arms lower than your heart.

If you suffer from SPD, keep a narrow stance with your knees above your hips or hardly wider.

For the benefits of these postures, see Chapter I Standing Postures.

Instructions: Sun-Salutations

1. Stand straight with the feet hip width apart (Mountain Pose) then take the hands to the heart centre. Inhale raising the arms up above the head, exhale swinging the arms down to the sides and keeping the knees bent, release the head and roll down (Forward Bend).

2. Inhale walking the hands away from you towards the front of the mat, exhale pressing the weight back and the heels down, stretching the spine and back of the legs (Down Dog).

3. Inhale releasing the knees to the floor, exhale releasing the head and round the back (Cat Stretch).

4. Inhale returning to All Fours (Neutral Cat), exhale placing the right foot forward outside the right hand to allow room for your bump. Inhale raising the arms up above the head hugging in your bump, exhale releasing the arms down. Take the finger tips to the floor inside the right hand.

Sun Salutations

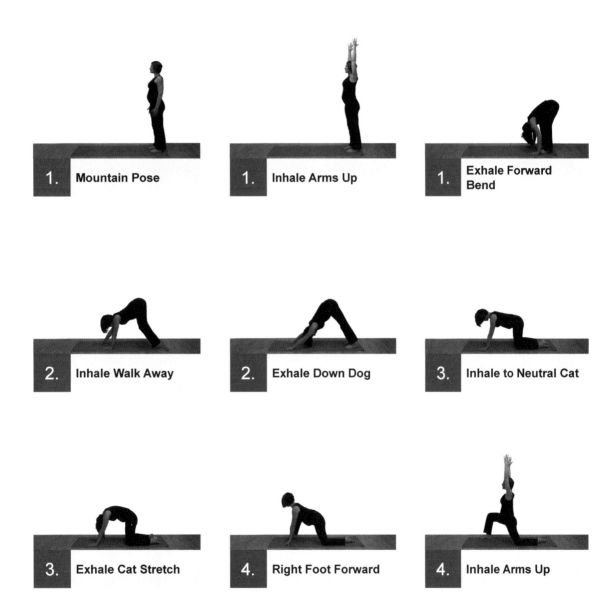

1. Mountain Pose

1. Inhale Arms Up

1. Exhale Forward Bend

2. Inhale Walk Away

2. Exhale Down Dog

3. Inhale to Neutral Cat

3. Exhale Cat Stretch

4. Right Foot Forward

4. Inhale Arms Up

Instructions: Sun-Salutations (Cont'd)

5. Ideally tuck the toes of the left foot under and straighten the left leg. Alternatively stay in the same position. Inhale leaning onto the left hand and lift the right arm up to the ceiling rotating the shoulder (Shoulder Rotation), exhale releasing the right hand to the floor.

6. Inhale sitting back placing the finger tips either side of the shins, straighten the right leg and flex the foot (Hamstring Stretch), exhale breathing through the stretch and stay for one additional breath.

7. Inhale coming back to All Fours (Neutral Cat), tuck the toes under, exhale pressing the weight back, straightening the legs and lifting the tailbone up to the ceiling (Down Dog).

8. Inhale walking the hands towards the feet, exhale releasing the head down (Forward Bend), knees bent and finger tips on the floor.

9. Inhale rolling up, then swing the arms above the head, exhale taking the hands down through the heart centre.

Repeat 1-9 to the left side and the whole sequence once for warm up to other sequences or several times as a stand-alone Standing Practice.

Sun Salutations (Cont'd)

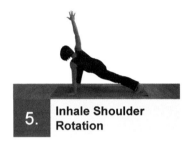

5. Inhale Shoulder Rotation

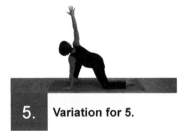

5. Variation for 5.

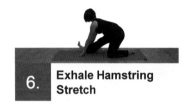

6. Exhale Hamstring Stretch

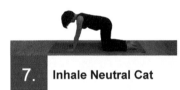

7. Inhale Neutral Cat

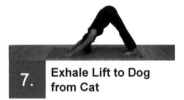

7. Exhale Lift to Dog from Cat

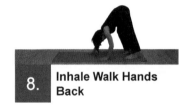

8. Inhale Walk Hands Back

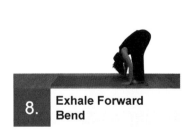

8. Exhale Forward Bend

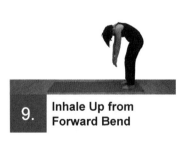

9. Inhale Up from Forward Bend

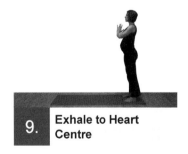

9. Exhale to Heart Centre

Instructions: Warrior Sequence

1. Stand straight with the feet hip width apart (Mountain). Inhale taking the feet and hands wide out to the sides keeping the feet parallel (Star), exhale lifting the muscles of the arms and legs, hug your bump in and look forward.

2. Inhale turning the right foot out 90 degrees and the left foot in 10 degrees, exhale.

3. Inhale sliding the left hand down the left thigh, turn the right palm up, lift the right arm to the ceiling and look up, exhale.

4. Inhale, exhale bending the right knee (Reverse Warrior).

5. Inhale moving the arms out to the sides, exhale keeping the right knee bent and look beyond the finger tips of the right hand, resisting with back leg and checking that the right knee is tracking the second toe and is at most above the ankle (Warrior II).

6. Inhale stretching out to the side through the right arm and take the right forearm to the right thigh, exhale taking the left hand to the hip, turn the navel to the front. Inhale lifting the left arm up to the ceiling (Side Angle), exhale.

7. Inhale straightening the right leg and right arm (Triangle), exhale, feel the lift through the chest keeping the legs strong.

8. Inhale coming up with the arms out to the sides, exhale lifting the muscles of the arms and legs.

9. Inhale rotating the feet forward and step in (Mountain).

Rest and repeat to the left side then repeat the whole sequence once or twice.

Warrior Sequence

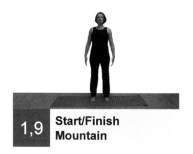

1,9 Start/Finish Mountain

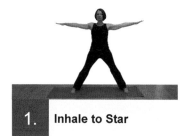

1. Inhale to Star

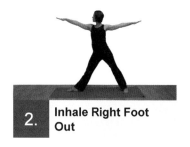

2. Inhale Right Foot Out

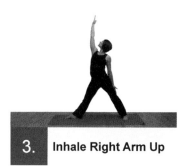

3. Inhale Right Arm Up

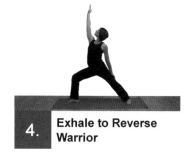

4. Exhale to Reverse Warrior

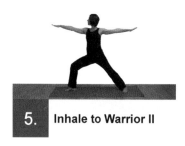

5. Inhale to Warrior II

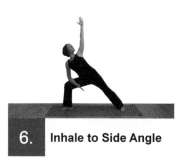

6. Inhale to Side Angle

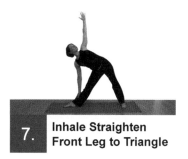

7. Inhale Straighten Front Leg to Triangle

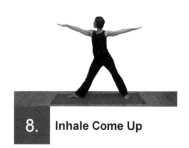

8. Inhale Come Up

Instructions: Lateral and Leg Stretches with Chair

1. Face the chair one foot away. Inhale raising the arms up above the head, exhale lowering the arms to the chair. Release the head down (Forward Bend). Press the feet into the floor and lift the muscles of the legs. Stay for 4 breaths.

2. Inhale stepping back until the legs are at 90 degrees with body, exhale extend the tailbone back (Down Dog). Feel the stretch through the sides of the rib cage. Press the feet down to lift the back of legs and keep tummy soft. Stay for 4 breaths

3. Inhale softening the knees, step in and roll up.

4. Inhale taking the left foot out 20 degrees and placing the right foot carefully on the chair (hold the wall or chair for balance). When steady, place the hands on the hips, square hips to chair and straightening the right leg, flex the foot. Inhale opening the chest, exhale folding forward slightly until you feel the strong stretch behind the right leg. Stay for 4 breaths.

5. Inhale coming up, bend the right leg foot flat on the chair, turn the left heel 70 degrees so the feet form a right angle. Place the right forearm inside the right bent knee.

6. Inhale taking the left arm to the side, reach up to the ceiling, exhale Side Bend to the right stretching the left side of the body. Stay for 2 breaths.

Carefully relax down, rest and repeat with the left foot forward. Repeat the whole sequence once or twice.

Lateral and Leg Stretches

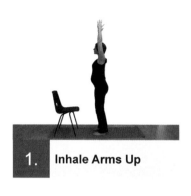

1. Inhale Arms Up

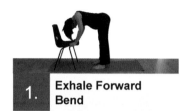

1. Exhale Forward Bend

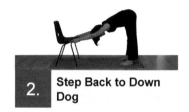

2. Step Back to Down Dog

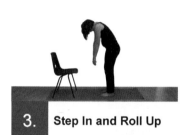

3. Step In and Roll Up

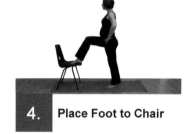

4. Place Foot to Chair

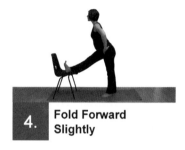

4. Fold Forward Slightly

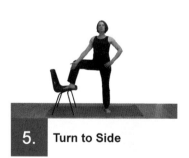

5. Turn to Side

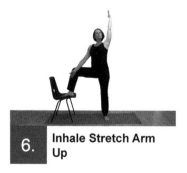

6. Inhale Stretch Arm Up

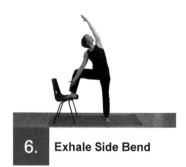

6. Exhale Side Bend

Instructions: Squats

1. Horse Stance Squat

   Start with the feet wide and pointing out. Inhale taking the arms up above the head, exhale taking the hands down through the heart centre, bend the knees into a low squat (Horse Stance). Hug your bump in and flatten the lower back. Stay for one breath. Inhale to come up. Repeat 4 times.

2. Side Angle Variation Squat

   Start with the feet wide and pointing out. Inhale taking the arms up above the head, exhale to Horse Stance. Place the right forearm inside the right thigh, inhale lifting the left arm up to the ceiling, exhale releasing the left arm to the inner left thigh (Side Angle Variation). Inhale raising the right arm up to the ceiling, exhale taking both hands to the heart centre. Stay for one breath and inhale to come up.

3. Lotus Flower Squat.

   Start with the feet wide and pointing out. Inhale taking the arms up and above the head, exhale to Horse Stance. Inhale moving the arms out to shoulder height (Lotus Flower Opens), exhale raising the arms up above the head (Lotus Flower Closes). Repeat 3 times then take the hands to the heart centre and inhale to come up.

4. Chair Pose

   Start with the feet parallel, hip width apart keeping your bump hugged in and the back flat throughout. Inhale softening the knees, exhale sitting on an imaginary chair and taking the arms up above the head. Hold for one breath and inhale to come up. Repeat 4 times.

Squats

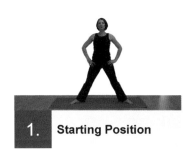

1.   Starting Position

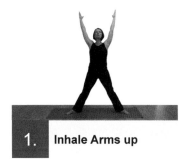

1.   Inhale Arms up

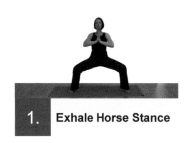

1.   Exhale Horse Stance

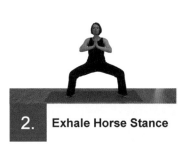

2.   Exhale Horse Stance

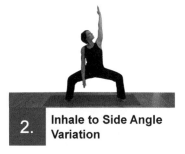

2.   Inhale to Side Angle Variation

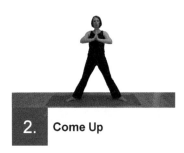

2.   Come Up

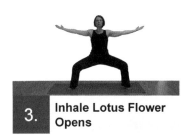

3.   Inhale Lotus Flower Opens

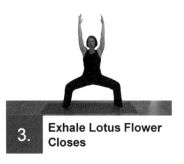

3.   Exhale Lotus Flower Closes

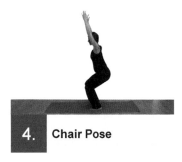

4.   Chair Pose

Instructions: Moon Salutations

1. Stand straight with the feet hip width apart (Mountain). Inhale raising the arms above the head, exhale Side Bend. Inhale moving back to centre, exhale Side Bend the other way.

2. Inhale taking the feet and arms out to the side with feet parallel (Star), exhale lifting the muscles of the legs and arms.

3. Inhale taking the right foot out 90 degrees, moving the left foot in 10 degrees, reach out side-ways through the right arm, exhale lowering the right hand to the right leg. Inhale lifting the left arm up to the ceiling (Triangle), exhale.

4. Take the hands to the hips, pivoting on the sole of the back foot and sliding the heel back, turn the hips to face the side of the mat. Inhale opening the chest, exhale lowering the body forward 30 degrees (Half Side Stretch). Feel the stretch in the back of the front leg.

5. Inhale coming up, exhale lowering the hands to the mat, slide the left leg back and drop the left knee to the floor (Lunge). Inhale taking the arms up above the head (Crescent Moon), exhale releasing hands to the mat (Lunge).

6. Inhale moving the feet parallel to the short side of the mat while the body is supported on the hands underneath the shoulders, exhale (Half Wide Leg Forward Bend).

Roll up and rest. Repeat to the other side. Repeat the complete sequence once or twice.

Moon Salutations

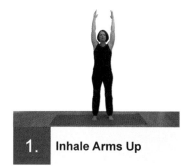

1. Inhale Arms Up

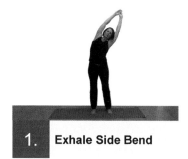

1. Exhale Side Bend

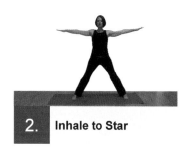

2. Inhale to Star

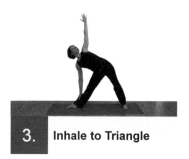

3. Inhale to Triangle

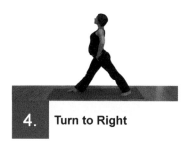

4. Turn to Right

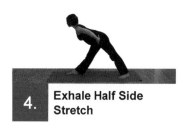

4. Exhale Half Side Stretch

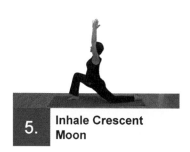

5. Inhale Crescent Moon

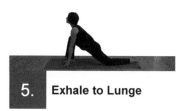

5. Exhale to Lunge

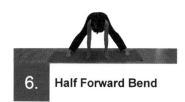

6. Half Forward Bend

Standing Sequences for Late Pregnancy (34 Weeks +)

In late pregnancy from 34 weeks you can still practice strong Standing Yoga postures which will continue to tone the arms and legs. However, choose to work with the support of a chair and take care not to overwork.

Instructions: Warrior Sequence with Chair

It is important to start sitting correctly on the chair. Stand with the feet wide and parallel and the chair right behind you. Take your right foot out 90 degrees and your left foot in. Lower to the chair so that your right sit bone only is supported. Your heels should be in a line and the back leg straight.

1. Inhale taking both arms up above the head as you turn to the right, turning your hips and back foot towards the short side of the mat, exhale lifting the muscles of the arms and legs, hug your bump in.

2. Inhale moving the arms forward, exhale pulling the left arm back at shoulder height (Bow and Arrow).

3. Inhale sliding the left hand down the left thigh, turn the right palm up and lift it up to the ceiling looking up (Reverse Warrior), exhale.

4. Inhale taking the arms out to the sides at shoulder height (Warrior II), exhale pressing the feet firmly into the floor look behind the finger tips of the right hand.

5. Inhale stretching out to the side through the right arm and take the right forearm to the right thigh, exhale taking the left hand to the hip, turn the navel to the front. Inhale lifting the left arm up above the head alongside the ear, exhale.

6. Come up centering yourself on the chair with the feet out in a squat position and bring the hands to the heart centre (Supported Horse Stance).

Rest and repeat to the left side. Repeat the whole sequence once or twice.

Warrior Sequence with Chair

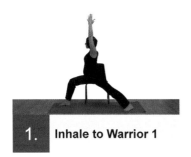

1. Inhale to Warrior 1

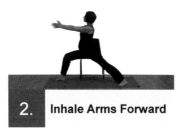

2. Inhale Arms Forward

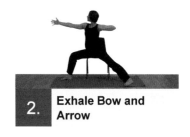

2. Exhale Bow and Arrow

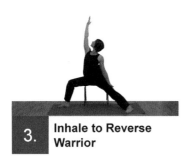

3. Inhale to Reverse Warrior

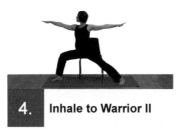

4. Inhale to Warrior II

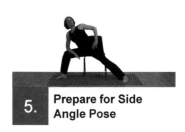

5. Prepare for Side Angle Pose

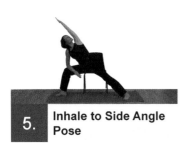

5. Inhale to Side Angle Pose

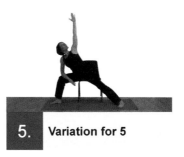

5. Variation for 5

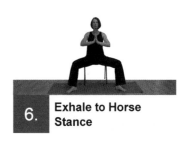

6. Exhale to Horse Stance

Instructions: Squats with Chair

Start in a standing position with the feet wide in front of the chair, feet pointing out to a comfortable position.

1. Supported Horse Stance Squat

   Inhale taking the arms up above the head, exhale taking the hands down through the heart centre and bend the knees into Horse Stance supported on the edge of the chair. Hug your bump in and flatten the lower back. Stay for one breath. Inhale to return to starting position. Repeat 4 times.

2. Supported Side Angle Variation Squat

   From starting position inhale taking the arms up above the head, exhale taking the hands down through the heart centre and bend the knees to Supported Horse Stance on the edge of the chair. Place the right forearm inside the right thigh, inhale lifting the left arm up to the ceiling (Side Angle Variation), exhale releasing the left arm to the inner left thigh. Inhale raising the right arm up to the ceiling, exhale taking both hands to the heart centre. Stay for one breath and inhale to starting position.

3. Supported Lotus Flower Squat.

   From starting position inhale taking the arms up above the head, exhale to Supported Horse Stance on the edge of the chair. Inhale moving the arms out to shoulder height (Lotus Flower Opens), exhale raising the arms up above the head (Lotus Flower Closes). Repeat 3 times then take the hands to the heart centre and inhale to return to starting position.

Squats with Chair

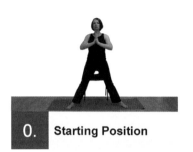

0.   **Starting Position**

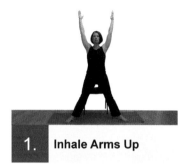

1.   **Inhale Arms Up**

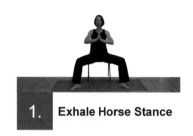

1.   **Exhale Horse Stance**

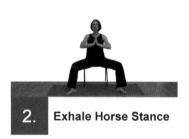

2.   **Exhale Horse Stance**

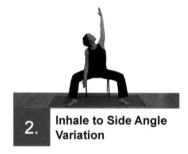

2.   **Inhale to Side Angle Variation**

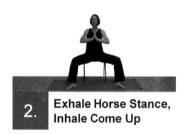

2.   **Exhale Horse Stance, Inhale Come Up**

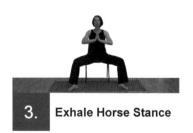

3.   **Exhale Horse Stance**

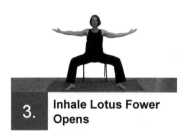

3.   **Inhale Lotus Fower Opens**

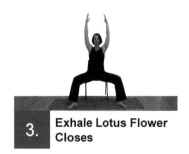

3.   **Exhale Lotus Flower Closes**

Instructions: Moon Salutations with Chair

1. Stand straight with the feet hip width apart (Mountain) and the Chair to your right side. Inhale raising the arms above the head, exhale Side Bend. Inhale moving back to centre, exhale Side Bend the other way.

2. Inhale taking the feet wide with feet parallel and the hands on the hips, exhale lifting the muscles of the legs.

3. Inhale taking the right foot out 90 degrees, moving the left foot in 10 degrees towards the chair. Lift the arms to shoulder height and reach out through the sides lowering the right hand to the chair in preparation for Triangle Pose. Rest the left hand on your hip as you lengthen the left side of the waist. Inhale lifting the left arm up to the ceiling (Triangle), exhale.

4. Pivoting on the sole of the back foot and sliding the heel back, turn the hips to face the side of the mat taking both hands to the chair (Half Side Stretch). Feel the stretch in the back of front leg as you lengthen the spine for one full breath.

5. Using the support of the chair, slide the left leg back and drop the left knee to the floor (Crescent Lunge). Take a full breath.

6. Inhale using the chair to come up, turn around and sit on the egde of the chair legs wide and feet turning out. Exhale lower the body between the legs, keeping hands on the thights for support if needed (Supported Forward Bend).

Roll up and rest. Repeat to the other side. Repeat the complete sequence once.

Moon Salutations with Chair

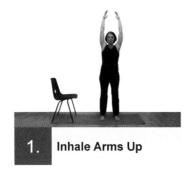

1. Inhale Arms Up

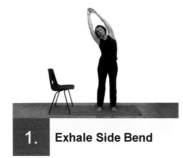

1. Exhale Side Bend

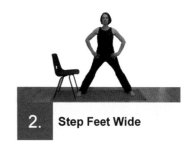

2. Step Feet Wide

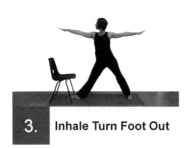

3. Inhale Turn Foot Out

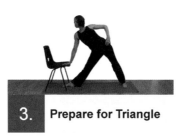

3. Prepare for Triangle

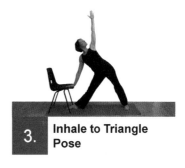

3. Inhale to Triangle Pose

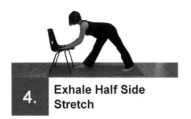

4. Exhale Half Side Stretch

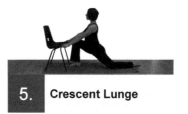

5. Crescent Lunge

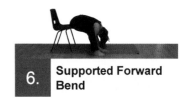

6. Supported Forward Bend

Final Floor Postures

These postures aim to close the Yoga practice, calming the mind prior to the Relaxation. They can be practiced all the way through your pregnancy. If you are suffering from pelvic pain and in particular Symphysis Pubis Pain, keep your knees in front of your hips at all times and avoid taking the knees out wide. For the benefits of postures see Chapter I.

Instructions: One-Leg Stretches with Belt

1. From simple cross-legged (Neutral) position open the right leg out to the side with the left foot resting towards the inner right thigh.

2. Turn towards the right leg, sit straight and flex the foot (toes to ceiling). Place the belt around the toe joints and lift up from the sit bones through the crown of the head, flexing the foot. Stay for 7-9 breaths.

3. Take the belt into the right hand, turn towards the left shoulder and extend the left arm back (Open Twist). Stay for 2 or 3 breaths. Inhale lifting the left arm up above the head and look up. Stay for 2 breaths.

4. Release the left hand to the left hip and drop the belt. Inhale raising the right arm up to the ceiling and stretch. Stay for 2 breaths.

5. Exhale releasing the right arm down, sliding the back of the right forearm to inside the right leg. Inhale raising the left arm up to the ceiling above the head, exhale Side Bend to the right. Feel the stretch to the back of the left waist.

Repeat to the other side.

One-Leg Stretches with Belt

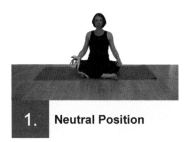

1. Neutral Position

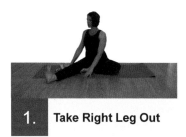

1. Take Right Leg Out

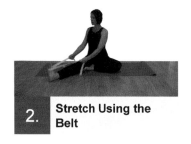

2. Stretch Using the Belt

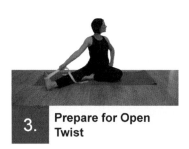

3. Prepare for Open Twist

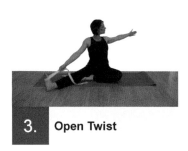

3. Open Twist

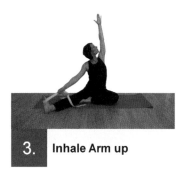

3. Inhale Arm up

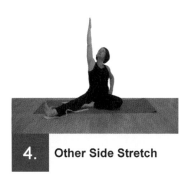

4. Other Side Stretch

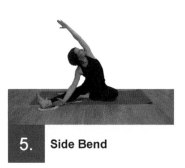

5. Side Bend

Instructions: Wide Leg Stretches to Forward Bend

1. From simple cross-legged (Neutral) position, open both legs out to the sides with the hands behind the sit bones for support. Keep well within your normal range of movement.

2. Bring the hands to the front, lift through the spine pressing down through the sit bones. Flex the feet, extending through the heels and press the thighs down. Stay for 5 breaths. Alternatively come down to the elbows without overstretching (Variation).

3. Move the hands to the right and reach up through the crown of the head pressing the thighs down. Stay for 5 breaths.

4. Inhale raising the left arm up to the ceiling and stretch using the back of the right hand against the inner right leg for leverage. Stay for one breath.

5. Exhale releasing the left hand to the left hip. Inhale raising the right arm up to the ceiling. Look up. Repeat 3-5 to the other side.

6. Bring the legs carefully together. Cross the legs and take the left hand to outside the right knee. Place the right hand finger tips behind you (Simple Cross-Legged Twist). Inhale reaching up, exhale turning the head to the right. Repeat to the other side.

7. Bring the soles of the feet together in a wide diamond shape, feet away from you. Slide the hands under the ankles to cup the feet and release the head down folding forward. Concentrate on the breath. Stay for 7 breaths.

Wide Leg Stretches to Forward Bend

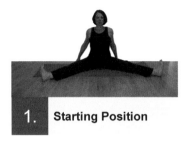

1. Starting Position

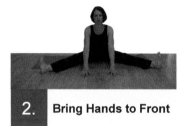

2. Bring Hands to Front

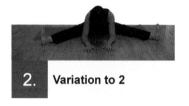

2. Variation to 2

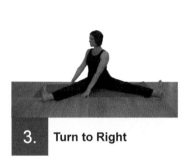

3. Turn to Right

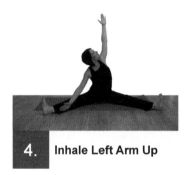

4. Inhale Left Arm Up

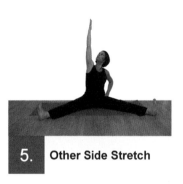

5. Other Side Stretch

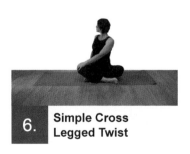

6. Simple Cross Legged Twist

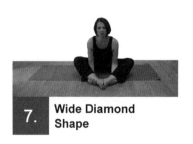

7. Wide Diamond Shape

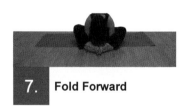

7. Fold Forward

Instructions: Pelvis Tilts

1. From simple cross-legged (Neutral) position rock from side to side on the sit bones (Rocking).

2. Draw circles with the body in one direction around the sit bones, change direction and draw the figure eight (Rolling). This works the hip and pelvis joints.

3. Place both feet flat on the floor in front of the hips using the hands around the knees for support. Inhale tilting the pelvis forward and using the hands for leverage expand the body upwards, exhale tucking the tailbone under, stretch the spine in a C shape. (Pelvic Tilt). Repeat 5 times.

4. Cross the left leg under and press the right elbow to inside the right knee. Take the left finger tips behind you. Inhale lifting up through the spine, exhale turning the head to the left (Open Twist). Repeat to the other side.

5. Place a block or chair in front of you. Cross the legs and release the head to the side onto the block. Relax the arms and hands (Forward Bend). Stay for 9 breaths. Use the hands to sit up.

Pelvis Tilts

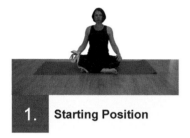

1. Starting Position

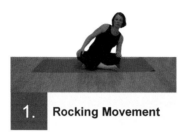

1. Rocking Movement

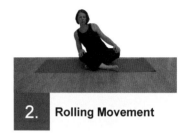

2. Rolling Movement

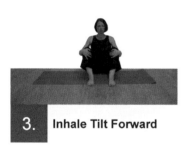

3. Inhale Tilt Forward

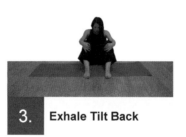

3. Exhale Tilt Back

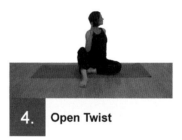

4. Open Twist

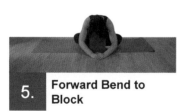

5. Forward Bend to Block

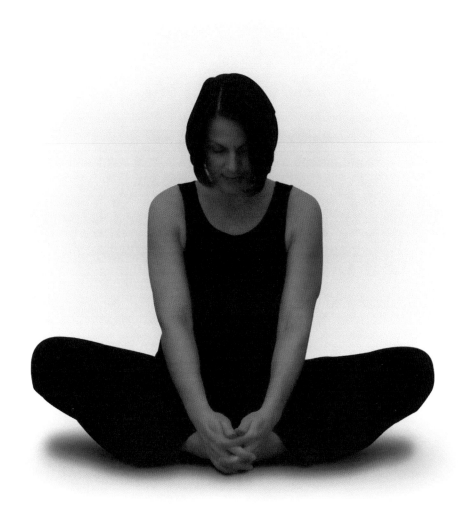

Chapter III
Relaxation

You can practice Relaxation all the way through your pregnancy.

Start as soon as you know you are pregnant. In the first trimester the development of your baby is truly amazing and demanding and Relaxation will really help you get the extra rest you will need.

In your trimester II and III you will continue to use the Relaxation time to rest and relax. Also you can truly start a Meditation practice helping you to connect with your baby and preparing you for childbirth.

Relaxation Postures and How to Practice

The Visualisation texts start with a Breathing Exercise which is an excellent way to centre yourself and prepare you for Relaxation. You will need to set aside a minimum of 20 minutes of your time to allow for the complete Relaxation practice. Note that you may want to relax and rest further at the end of the practice.

To prepare record each of the following texts so that you can play them back to yourself during the Relaxation. Take care to speak slowly and include a silent breath or two where the text is marked by several dots.

First you will need to build an incline of 30-45 degrees to prevent putting too much pressure on the main arteries (vena cava) running along the lower back. If you have got Yoga equipment available use two bolsters in a cross or one bolster supported over 4 blocks as pictured below. Alternatively you can form a bolster by rolling a large blanket and elevate it using a pile of cushions or stacked blankets.

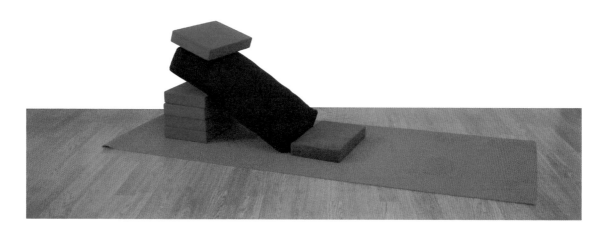

Have a block or rolled blanket on hand to elevate the head a little further as needed and perhaps some additional blocks or rolled blankets to support the arms and knees.

Supported Reclined Butterfly Pose

This is a wonderfully relaxing posture which helps to loosen and relax the pelvis and hips, an area where we hold a lot of tension. Be sure to support the knees completely so that there is no stretch felt. The groin area and tummy must remain soft for you to be able to completely relax.

Should the arms pull on the shoulders support the elbows and forearms on additional height using a block, rolled blankets or large books.

Start with practicing this posture for a few minutes and build up to 20 minutes. Choose this Pose in particular when working with the Visualisation texts that build confidence for labour (Enhance Your Emotional Strength and Visualisation for Labour Preparation).

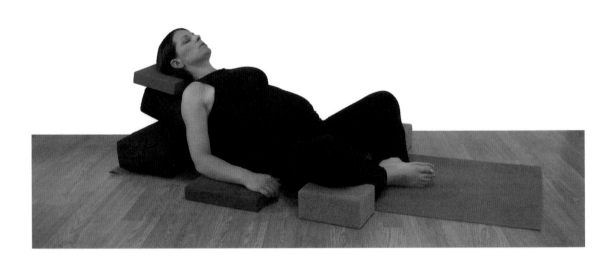

Supported Savasana Pose

Savasana is the traditional pose for Yoga Relaxation and is used throughout the world at the end of every Yoga class.

During Relaxation time we engage the parasympathetic side of the nervous system. This is the part that is normally more active during rest and sleep. It is responsible for helping to slow down our body activity and neutralise stress and the effect of stress on the body.

On the physical side, it is critical to help the body relax and the muscles to heal and repair. On the mental side, it is providing us with some time when the brain and agitation of the mind is set aside. On the emotional side, it is a gift from yourself to allow you to rest and relax.

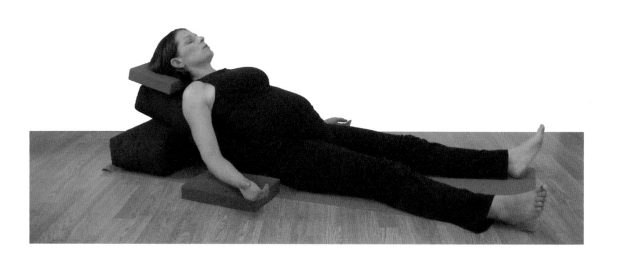

As with the previous Pose, plan for a 30-45 degrees incline using bolsters, blankets or pillows, a cushion for the head and some height for the elbows and forearms.

Choose the Yoga Nidra text for this position or perhaps Enhance Your Emotional Bond with emphasis on the openness of the chest, lifting the heart centre.

A Posture For When Time Is Short

If you only have 5 minutes sit on a cushion cross-legged against a wall for support and support the knees as needed so you can sit straight but are comfortable. Practice the initial Breathing Exercise for 5 minutes.

If you find that you have more time continue with the complete Relaxation routine. You can continue to sit up or use one of the preceding Relaxation Postures. Alternatively lie down on your left side, placing a cushion under the head and between the knees.

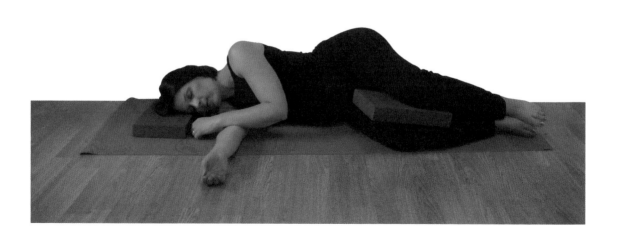

Visualisation Texts: Overview

Once you are comfortable you are ready to start your practice. You can choose from the following Visualisation and Relaxation Exercises. They will guide you through the Relaxation.

- Yoga Nidra Relaxation. Yoga Nidra is a technique used in Yoga classes, Meditation classes and other therapies. The text guides you through all parts of the body, encouraging you to mentally and physically release tension.

- Enhance Your Emotional Strength. This Relaxation text leads you to meditate on the energy centre called the Base Chakra at the base of the spine. This energy centre is associated with the qualities of strength, stability and feeling secure and grounded. These are the emotions that help neutralise fear and anxiety.

- Building Confidence. This Relaxation Exercise is for building a visualisation of a special place where a feeling of peace and tranquillity, contentment and confidence may be experienced. It encourages you to imagine your baby is safe, comfortable and secure inside your body. This place will be an imaginary area that you can visualise and recall whenever you need it to help calm and relax your mind and body.

- Enhance Your Emotional Bond. This is a Meditation Exercise, on the heart centre filling it with the feeling of love and joy and sharing this feeling of well being with your baby. This practice will help enhance your sense of connection with your baby. You can sit up or recline in Savasana keeping one hand on your heart and the other on your bump.

- Light As A Feather. This Visualisation Exercise feels like a therapeutic treatment particularly suited in late pregnancy. It is designed to make you feel light, weighless and spacious. Enjoy.

- Visualisation for Labour Preparation. This Relaxation Exercise uses the Earth Energy or Wave Breathing technique. This technique is invaluable during contractions to help focus the mind away from the pain. It also includes a complementary Breathing technique which helps recuperation between contractions.

Practice guided Meditation or Relaxation as often as possible to help you effectively relax during labour. Visualisation and Relaxation are techniques that need rehearsing: the more you practice, the more effective they will become.

All guided Relaxation exercises are recorded by Laurence as part of her on-line classes at www.pregnancyyogaclasses.com/book (Menu Meditation and Final Relaxation)

Visualisation Texts to Record and Practice

Try to record each of the following texts so that you can play them back to yourself during Relaxation. Speak slowly taking a silent breath or two where the text is marked by several dots thereby allowing you to let go with the suggestions.

Yoga Nidra Relaxation

In this Relaxation Exercise you are scanning each body part in turn, from your toes to your head, to mentally and physically release tension. Make sure you are lying comfortably on your support, head and arms supported.

This is the most important time of your practice when you are giving yourself a chance to rest and let go, letting the body heal and repair and taking an opportunity to connect with yourself and your baby.

Concentrate on your breathing, listening to the sound of your breath..... For the next few breaths count to four on the inhale and four on the exhale.....

Now you can relax and let go, letting the feet flop gently to the sides...... Feel the weight of the right heel sinking into the floor..... and the left..... Let the right calf relax onto the floor..... and the left.....

Now focusing on the right thigh..... softly giving in, heavy on the mat..... and the left, rolling outwards resting on the floor.....

Feel the weight of the buttocks, pelvis and hips sinking into the floor..... the back spreading..... feel the space it takes on the support up the spine and to the shoulders..... release the shoulders open and free, the arms supported..... Feel as if you are melting into the floor now although completely supported..... Tuck the chin in slightly lengthening the neck.....

Relax the muscles of the face and jaw.... feel the lips soften into a contented smile..... feel all the muscles round the eyes soften and the eyes sink back into their sockets.....

Release across the forehead and the top of the head..... feel the scalp releasing down the back of the head.....

You are sinking into a deep state of Relaxation now.....

Gently take your awareness to your Breathing..... follow the sound of your breath..... feel your breath filling your tummy and gently massaging your baby as your abdomen softens and relaxes to the wave like motion of the breath..... Each breath is connecting you to your baby, exchanging life force and energy and also calming and soothing, rocking your baby as you inhale and exhale.....

As you are approaching the end of the Relaxation take a few minutes to clear your mind of any thoughts, remaining quietly in silence..... If you choose to fall asleep that will be fine and when you are ready to come out of this state bring your attention back to the room, letting all of your senses awaken..... become aware of the sounds in the room..... feel the touch of your clothes on your skin..... take a deep breath.

Make small movements with your hands and feet..... sit up using your arms and hands for support to avoid straining any part of your lower back or the abdomen.

Enhance Your Emotional Strength

In this Meditation you are using a Visualisation to feel grounded, stable and strong and confident that you will know how to give birth. It will give you time to rest and nurture yourself and in turn your baby.

Now you can relax and let go, taking your awareness to your Breathing, listening to the sound of your breath, its pace and rhythm..... focus on the air passing in and out of the nostrils..... notice the temperature of the air..... cooler as you breathe in..... warmer as you breathe out..... Try to trace the flow of the air inside your body..... Passing into the throat..... the ribcage and the chest..... the abdomen.....

Now moving your awareness to the contact of your body with the floor or support..... Feel the sit bones pressing evenly on the floor..... imagine the earth below you..... the rocks..... the solid ground.....

With each inhale visualise the Earth Energy moving up the front of your body and over your head..... and with the exhale down your back and into the ground..... Continue this Visualisation, imagining a loop of energy, up the front of your body as you inhale and down the back of your body as you exhale..... now try to lengthen the exhale .....

Now concentrate on the base of your spine and feel a warming sensation..... Visualise the colour red. When meditating on the Energy Centre at the base of the spine we visualise the colour red..... Now see the colour red spreading around the base of the spine and pelvis..... the intensity of the colour and the warming sensation get stronger with each breath you take..... it spreads towards the legs..... extends down into the floor..... it connects the pelvis and legs to the floor..... now let the colour and warmth spread up all round your lower back.....

As you are connected into the earth, draw from the earth, the qualities of strength, stability and safety..... experience feeling strong and confident.....

My body will know how to give birth..... Now repeat to yourself 'I have no fear'.

As you are approaching the end of the Relaxation take a few minutes to clear your mind of any thoughts, remaining quietly in silence..... When you are ready to come out of this state bring your attention back to the room, letting your awareness expand beyond the space you are taking up on the floor..... become aware of the sounds in the room..... feel the touch of your clothes on your skin..... take a deep breath.

Make small movements with your hands and feet..... Sit up using your arms and hands for support to avoid straining any part of your lower back or the abdomen.

Building Confidence

Begin by taking a moment to feel completely relaxed. Whether sitting up or lying down on your support close the eyes and allow yourself to completely let go and relax.

This is the most important part of your Yoga practice when you are giving yourself the opportunity to rest and relax.

Now take your awareness to your Breathing listening to the sound of your breath..... notice the pace of your breath..... its rhythm..... For the next few breaths count to four on the inhale and four on the exhale.... If your mind wanders start the counting again....

Continue to breathe slowly, breathe easy..... let the rate of your breathing become free as your body relaxes.

You are now feeling deeply relaxed..... and calm.....

Visualise a special place where you can completely relax..... a place where no-one else can go..... just you and your baby..... it may be indoors..... outdoors..... or even a special place within your heart..... This is a haven where you have no worries, cares or concerns..... this place gives you a feeling of total calm..... peaceful and warm..... you can just relax and enjoy being..... happy and content.....

What will this wonderful place need to be like for you to feel calm and relaxed?..... Look around you..... what colours are there..... what sounds..... imagine any tastes or smells..... any sense of touch it holds..... how warm the air is..... Imagine if you are doing anything..... or maybe you are just content being there.....

Enjoy your special place for a few moments more..... see if you can hold in your mind the picture of your special place, how it feels..... now store this feeling in your heart.

Now keep your focus on your heart.... experience a deep sense of peace and tranquillity..... It swirls around your heart..... filling the heart area..... Imagine it is now spreading from your heart to your navel..... spreading and radiating..... sharing this sense of well being with your baby..... the placenta is strong..... the amniotic fluid is plentiful and rich in nutrients..... your baby's heart rate is strong and steady and baby is safe, comfortable and secure inside.....

Feel that you can return to this place in your mind whenever you feel anxious and need to calm yourself..... You can picture your special place to allow yourself to deeply relax and build the confidence that all is well and will go well.

As you are approaching the end of the Relaxation take a few minutes to clear your mind of any thoughts, remaining quietly in silence..... When you are ready to come out of this state bring your attention back to the room, letting your awareness expand beyond the mat..... become aware of the sounds in the room..... feel the touch of your clothes on your skin..... take a deep breath.

Make small movements with your hands and feet..... Sit up using your arms and hands for support to avoid straining any part of your lower back or the abdomen.

Enhance Your Emotional Bond

This Meditation guides you to create a Visualisation to help you feel open and loving and able to receive and experience the love which you can share with you baby. It enhances your connection with your baby through this love.

Practice this meditation sitting up with the right hand on your chest and the left hand on your bump and baby or supported at 30- 45 degree on a couple of bolsters, in supported Savasana.

Now is time to relax and let go..... this is the most important part of your practice when you give yourself a chance to rest..... taking this time aside to nurture yourself and in turn your baby.

Now take your awareness to your Breathing, listening to the sound of your breath..... its pace and rhythm..... focus on the air passing in and out of the nostrils..... notice the temperature of the air..... cooler as you breathe in..... warmer as you breathe out..... Try to trace the flow of the air inside your body..... Passing into the throat..... the ribcage and chest..... the abdomen.....

Now follow to the movement of the body as you breathe..... Notice the subtle movement of the chest and rib cage,..... rising on the inhale and relaxing down on the exhale..... feel the movement of your tummy..... as you inhale into the tummy..... feel the air gently massaging your baby..... as you exhale..... release any tension..... notice the tummy gently releasing towards the spine.....

Gradually prepare to take deeper breaths..... Inhale slowly and deeply into the tummy, filling the abdomen like a balloon..... release all the air exhaling long and slow..... release all the tension with the breath..... and again.... inhale..... exhale..... inhale..... exhale.....

Now concentrate on your heart centre..... focus on the heart and feel the space around the heart chamber..... In Yoga, when meditating on the Heart

Centre, the colour green is visualised..... With each breath imagine the colour green gently bathing the heart and penetrating any space around it..... feel the space..... the ease with which you are able to breathe.....

Now imagine you are breathing in love and kindness..... experience how it feels..... comforting..... secure..... content..... allow your lips to gently smile..... As you breathe in, experience love into your heart..... as you breathe out, transfer this feeling of love to your baby..... Inhale into your right hand..... transfer to your left hand and your baby..... Feel the connection you are making with your baby,..... send a message of love to your baby.

As you are approaching the end of the Relaxation, slowly take your attention back to your breathing,..... observe the pace and sound of the breath..... take a few minutes to clear your mind of any thoughts, remaining quietly in silence.....

When you are ready to come out of this state bring your attention back to the room, letting your awareness expand beyond the space you are taking up on the floor..... become aware of the sounds in the room and the light streaming through the closed eye lids..... feel the touch of your clothes on your skin..... take a deep breath letting the oxygen revitalise the body.

Make small movements with your hands and feet..... take the hands into the heart centre.....

Light As A Feather

This Relaxation Exercise is a calming Visualisation that will guide you to imagine yourself feeling light, spacious and weightless.

Settle yourself down either on your left side, supported by blocks and cushions or in a reclined position at a 30-45 degree angle; completely comfortable and supported.

Now it is time to relax and let go, taking this time just for yourself and your baby. As you are relaxing, you are engaging the parasympathetic side of your nervous system which is its healing part, normally mostly active during sleep.

First allow a feeling of Relaxation to begin..... Starting from the top of the head, feel it deepen with each breath you take..... flowing through your hair..... now your face and ears..... now spreading to your neck..... your shoulders releasing towards the floor..... the softness now reaching your arms and hands.....

Move your awareness to your chest and upper back and feel them relaxing..... let the feeling of Relaxation flow through the middle of your back to your tummy..... and on to the base of your spine..... Relax your hips and pelvis..... let the relaxation travel through your thighs..... down your knees..... all the way to your feet and toes.....

Take a deep breath in..... breathe out any remaining tension.....

You are now feeling deeply relaxed and calm..... ready to visualise.....

Imagine that you are lying on a soft and comfortable bed of feathers..... Feel the surface beneath you soften yet it supports you giving a feeling of complete protection.....

The air is warm..... the feathers are slowly rising on the warm air, carrying you with them..... it is just as if you are floating on air..... now rising up and away..... you float on..... up into a blue and sunny sky..... warm, cosy and safe.

Feel the feathers touching each part of your body..... how comfortable it feels..... how soothing.

You are up in the bright clean air..... it is so clean..... your breathing is easier, calmer..... Take a deep breath in..... a slow breath out..... feel the space in your chest, how light and open it feels.

Your feathers are gently swaying with the breeze..... a warm, balmy breeze..... drifting up, up and away..... carrying you, so light and freed from the weight of your body..... it feels so comfortable and easy.....

Looking all around you see the beautiful sky..... the white fluffy clouds..... close enough to touch..... you float through them..... feel the mist on your cheeks as you rise.....

The sun shines through the clouds, lighting your feathers to give a bright glow..... this light is now penetrating every cell in your body..... a healing light, naturally cleansing and removing any toxins from your body..... protecting your baby with its warm, incandescent glow..... encouraging your baby to grow strong and well.....

As you are approaching the end of the Relaxation take a moment to clear your mind of any thoughts, remaining quietly in silence for the next few minutes or so.....

When you are ready to come out, take your attention back into the room, letting all of your senses awaken. Become aware of the sounds around you..... feel the contact of your clothes on your skin..... take a deep breath in letting the oxygen revitalise the body..... Make small movements with the hands and feet..... come up to sitting using the arms and hands to avoid straining any part of the lower back or the abdomen.

Visualisation for Labour Preparation

This Relaxation Exercise creates a Visualisation to help you between and through your contractions during labour by drawing on earth energy with Wave Breathing. This technique is invaluable during contractions to help focus the mind away from the pain. It also includes a complementary Breathing technique which helps recuperation between contractions.

First, make sure that you are sitting comfortably in a cross-legged position, resting against a wall or pillows with your knees supported by blocks and cushions or in a reclined position at a 30-45 degree angle completely comfortable and supported.

Now it is time to relax and let go. This is the most important part of your practice when you are taking some time to nurture yourself and therefore your baby.

Allow your body to relax into the support..... feeling completely supported and comfortable.....

Take your awareness to your Breathing..... Feel the movement through the body like a wave moving up and down to the rhythm of your breath..... Inhaling..... and exhaling..... slowly letting any tension out of the body.....

Now take your attention to the pelvis..... resting on the floor or the support..... imagine the contact with the earth..... As you breathe in, imagine you are breathing in the Earth Energy up through the front of the body..... and over the crown of the head..... as you breathe out, the energy moves down the back of the body and back into the earth..... Feel a wave of Relaxation flowing up from the pelvis to the top of the head as you inhale ..... and down the back of the body as you exhale..... The Earth Energy is bringing life force through the front of the body and releasing any tension as you exhale down the back of the body.....

You are fully relaxed now, you can start to visualise..... Imagine you are on a warm golden beach close to the sea..... Take a moment to picture this in your mind.....

You walk closer to the waves, and feel the sand becoming cooler and firmer. You sit down..... listening to the coming and going of the waves.....you find your breath is in time with the movement of the waves..... Inhale..... your breath comes up as the waves move in towards the shore, over the crown of the head as the waves break, and down your back as you exhale the waves receding towards the sea..... Continue for a few breaths.....

You find yourself deeply relaxed, ready to give birth, fully confident your body will know how to give birth.....

As a contraction comes in like a wave..... helping to open the cervix..... breathe in through the front of the body..... breathe out through the back of the body..... focus on the wave breathing ..... three breaths is all it takes for every contraction..... each breath is taking you closer,..... don't get concerned by the intensity..... your body is working perfectly..... let your body open..... surrender to the power of the contraction..... it is helping you.....bringing your baby closer with each breath.....

The contraction has subsided..... you find yourself back on your beach..... feel the relief of this moment..... a break for you and your baby..... inhale deeply and slowly into the tummy..... your breath is soothing your baby after the storm..... exhale slowly..... your breath is reassuring your baby that all is well..... inhale..... exhale..... inhale..... exhale...... you both need this recuperation time to prepare for the next contraction..... you are both ready.....

As you are approaching the end of the Relaxation, slowly take your attention back to your breathing,..... observe the pace and sound of the breath..... take a few minutes to clear your mind of any thoughts, remaining quietly in silence.....

When you are ready to come out of this state bring your attention back to the room, letting your awareness expand beyond the space you are taking up on the floor..... become aware of the sounds in the room and the light streaming through the closed eye lids..... feel the touch of your clothes on your skin..... take a deep breath letting the oxygen revitalise the body.....

Make small movements with your hands and feet.....

If lying down, sit up using your arms and hands for support to avoid straining any part of your lower back or the abdomen.

Thank you

Thank you for your interest and I really hope that some of this information will be helpful to you. I always felt that the information about how the brain and hormones work would really have helped me during my first labour if only I had known.

This understanding has re-ascertained the role of Breathing and Relaxation not only for birthing but also in various parts of my life and yoga practice. As for your practice and preparation for your birth select one of two Breathing and Visualisation exercises that work best for you and practice them until they become second nature so that no thinking is required during labour.

Do keep in touch, you can email me and I look forward to hearing your wonderful news in due time.

Namaste

Acknowledgements

Thank you all for making this possible. First of all my Teachers who have inspired me and given me the confidence to believe that I too could help and teach others. Also I am indebted to my pregnant students who are a constant source of inspiration and learning and the new mothers whose birth stories and testimonies are a credit to women's inner power and confirm the benefits of Yoga Breathing practices.

Special thanks go to my family who have been encouraging me. In particular my husband Phillip who has motivated and helped me in many ways and most importantly our beautiful daughter Luz whose arrival put me on this path and our second daughter Abigail who is portrayed as a bump on every picture in the book.

I would also like to warmly thank Marion Moldon who put her life on hold to edit the book and Lise Cairns who helped with the cover photos (Lise Cairns ©).

Laurence on the Internet

Laurence's on-line Pregnancy Yoga classes, claim your free class

www.pregnancyyogaclasses.com/book

Laurence's Pregnancy Yoga magazine, including interviews with the experts

www.Pregnancy-Yoga.Net

For Laurence's Yoga classes in Reigate and Redhill, Surrey, UK

www.Yogamoo.com

Connect with Laurence on Facebook

www.facebook.com/PregnancyYoga

Get Laurence's Tweets

www.twitter.com/yogamoo

View video samples

www.youtube.com/PregnancyYoga

Printed in Great
Britain
by Amazon

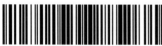